- Table of Conte

Bones Of The Skull
(Frontal View)

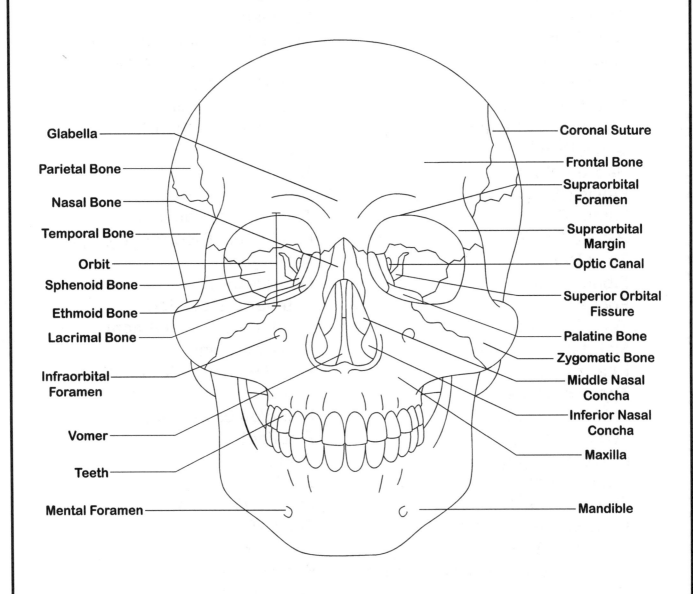

Glabella

Parietal Bone

Nasal Bone

Temporal Bone

Orbit

Sphenoid Bone

Ethmoid Bone

Lacrimal Bone

Infraorbital Foramen

Vomer

Teeth

Mental Foramen

Coronal Suture

Frontal Bone

Supraorbital Foramen

Supraorbital Margin

Optic Canal

Superior Orbital Fissure

Palatine Bone

Zygomatic Bone

Middle Nasal Concha

Inferior Nasal Concha

Maxilla

Mandible

Bones Of The Skull
(Lateral View)

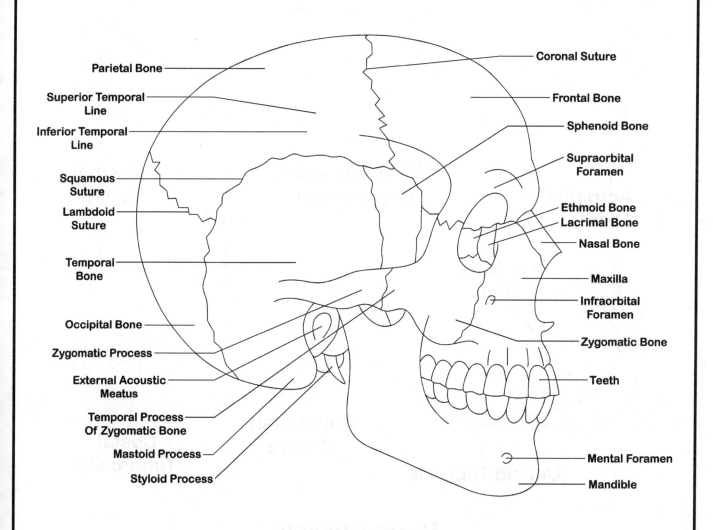

Parietal Bone

Superior Temporal Line

Inferior Temporal Line

Squamous Suture

Lambdoid Suture

Temporal Bone

Occipital Bone

Zygomatic Process

External Acoustic Meatus

Temporal Process Of Zygomatic Bone

Mastoid Process

Styloid Process

Coronal Suture

Frontal Bone

Sphenoid Bone

Supraorbital Foramen

Ethmoid Bone
Lacrimal Bone

Nasal Bone

Maxilla

Infraorbital Foramen

Zygomatic Bone

Teeth

Mental Foramen

Mandible

Clavicle

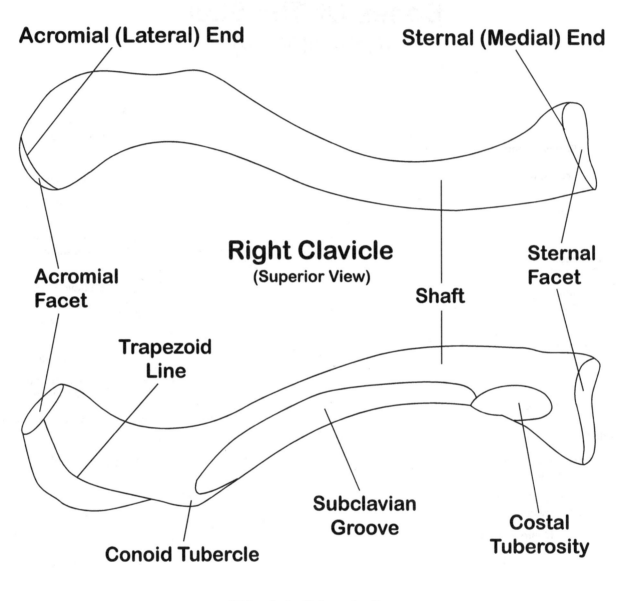

Acromial (Lateral) End

Sternal (Medial) End

Right Clavicle
(Superior View)

Acromial Facet

Sternal Facet

Shaft

Trapezoid Line

Subclavian Groove

Conoid Tubercle

Costal Tuberosity

Right Clavicle
(Inferior View)

Scapula

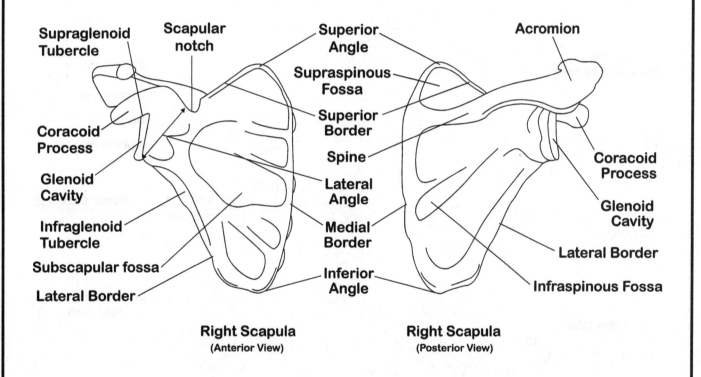

Supraglenoid Tubercle
Scapular notch
Superior Angle
Acromion
Supraspinous Fossa
Coracoid Process
Superior Border
Glenoid Cavity
Spine
Coracoid Process
Infraglenoid Tubercle
Lateral Angle
Glenoid Cavity
Subscapular fossa
Medial Border
Lateral Border
Lateral Border
Inferior Angle
Infraspinous Fossa

Right Scapula
(Anterior View)

Right Scapula
(Posterior View)

Rib Cage

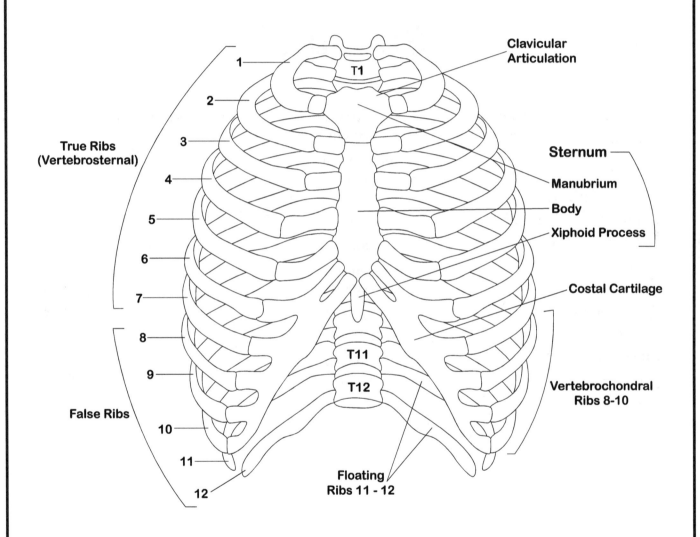

Clavicular
Articulation

T1

True Ribs
(Vertebrosternal)

Sternum

Manubrium

Body

Xiphoid Process

Costal Cartilage

T11

T12

Vertebrochondral
Ribs 8-10

False Ribs

Floating
Ribs 11 - 12

1
2
3
4
5
6
7
8
9
10
11
12

Sternum

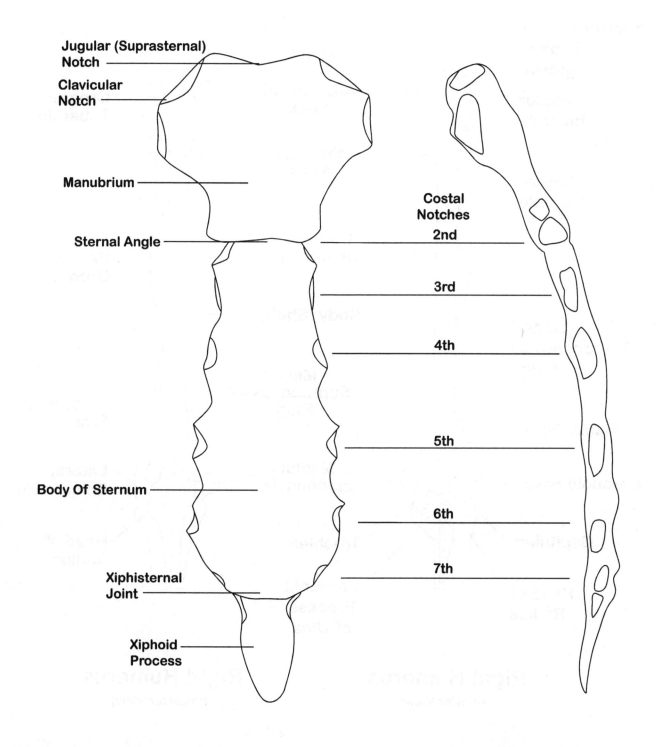

Jugular (Suprasternal) Notch

Clavicular Notch

Manubrium

Sternal Angle

Body Of Sternum

Xiphisternal Joint

Xiphoid Process

Costal Notches

2nd

3rd

4th

5th

6th

7th

Humerus

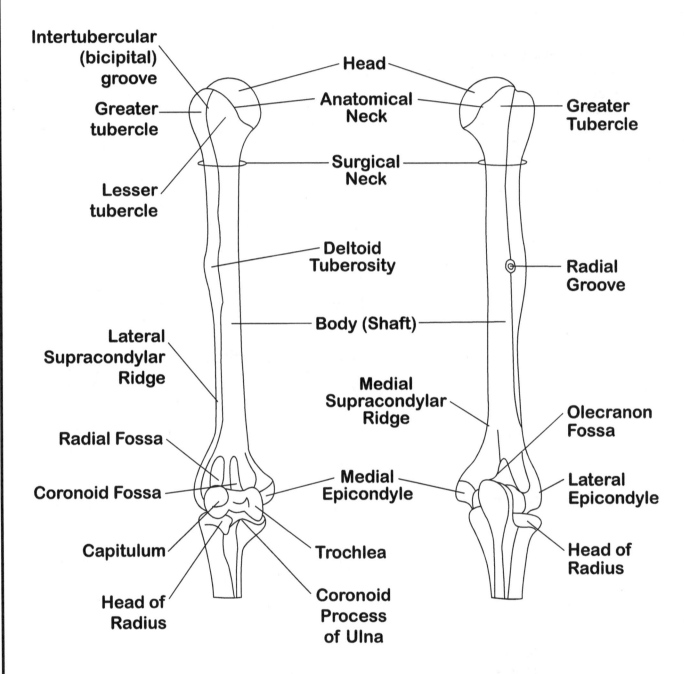

Intertubercular (bicipital) groove

Greater tubercle

Lesser tubercle

Head

Anatomical Neck

Surgical Neck

Deltoid Tuberosity

Body (Shaft)

Greater Tubercle

Radial Groove

Lateral Supracondylar Ridge

Radial Fossa

Coronoid Fossa

Capitulum

Head of Radius

Medial Supracondylar Ridge

Medial Epicondyle

Trochlea

Coronoid Process of Ulna

Olecranon Fossa

Lateral Epicondyle

Head of Radius

Right Humerus
(Anterior View)

Right Humerus
(Posterior View)

Radius

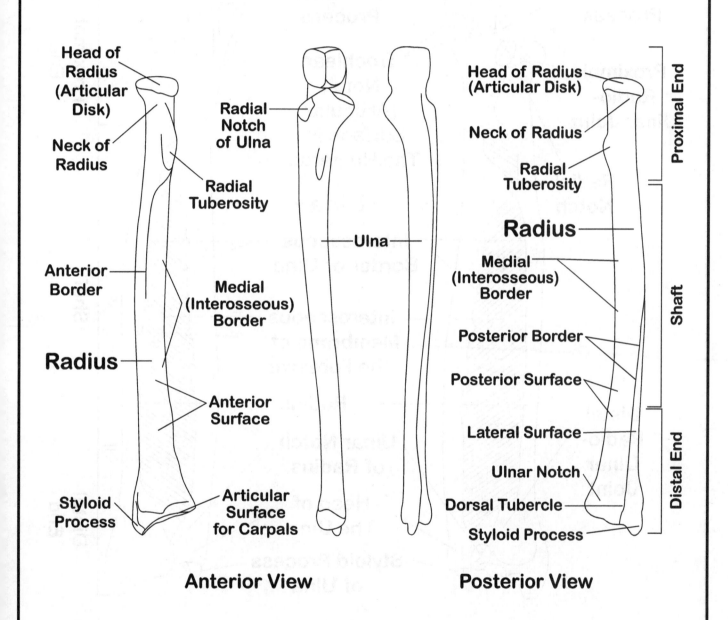

Head of Radius (Articular Disk)

Neck of Radius

Anterior Border

Radius

Styloid Process

Radial Notch of Ulna

Radial Tuberosity

Ulna

Medial (Interosseous) Border

Anterior Surface

Articular Surface for Carpals

Anterior View

Head of Radius (Articular Disk)

Neck of Radius

Radial Tuberosity

Radius

Medial (Interosseous) Border

Posterior Border

Posterior Surface

Lateral Surface

Ulnar Notch

Dorsal Tubercle

Styloid Process

Proximal End

Shaft

Distal End

Posterior View

Ulna

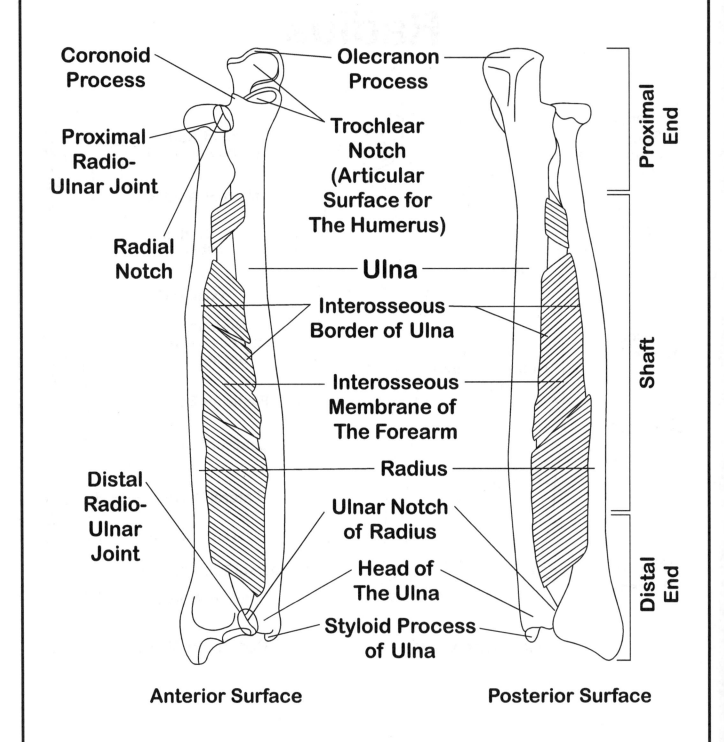

Coronoid Process

Olecranon Process

Proximal Radio-Ulnar Joint

Trochlear Notch (Articular Surface for The Humerus)

Radial Notch

Ulna

Interosseous Border of Ulna

Interosseous Membrane of The Forearm

Radius

Distal Radio-Ulnar Joint

Ulnar Notch of Radius

Head of The Ulna

Styloid Process of Ulna

Proximal End

Shaft

Distal End

Anterior Surface

Posterior Surface

Hand Bones

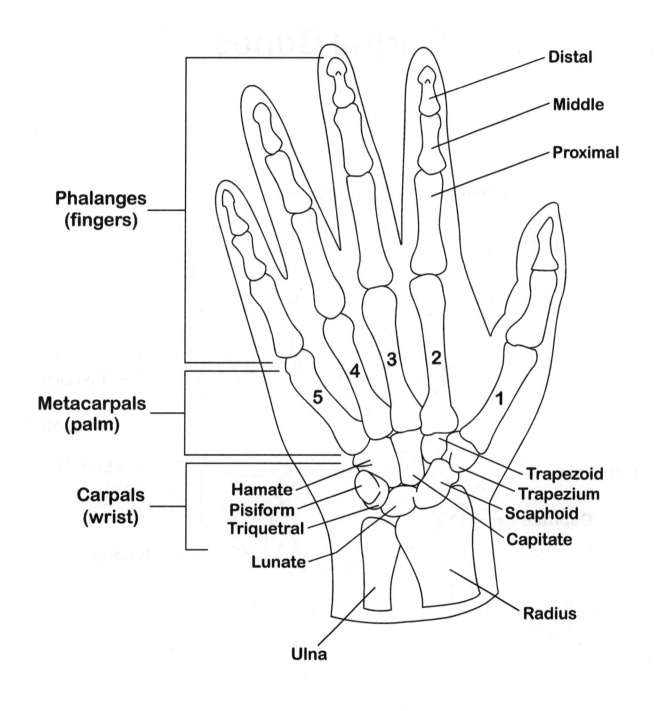

Carpal Bones

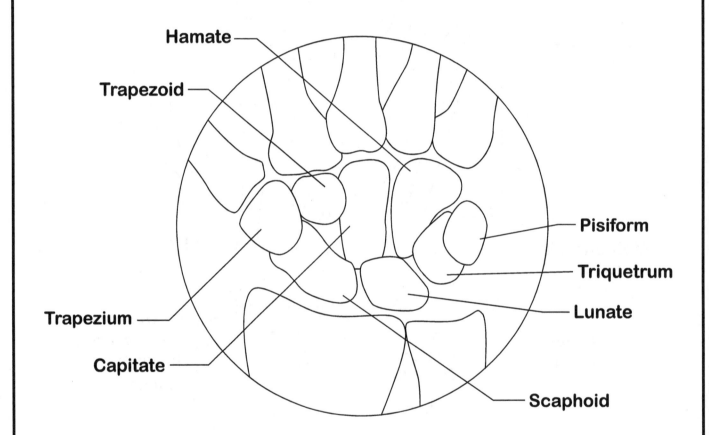

Metacarpal Bones

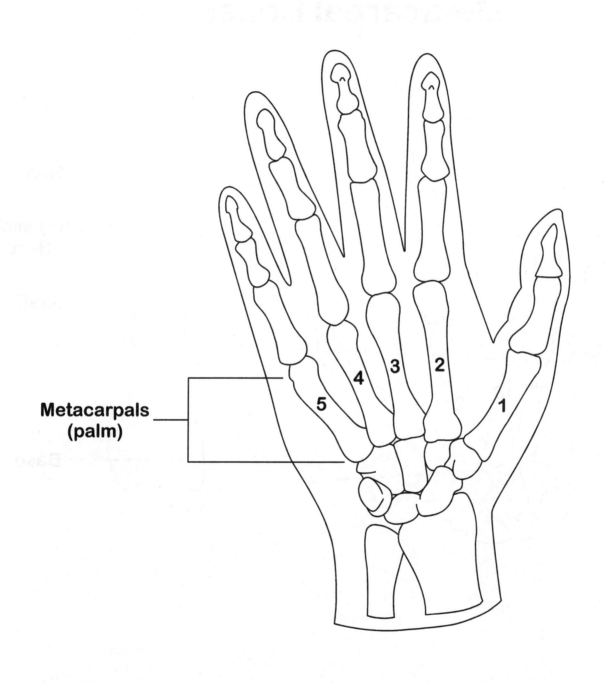

Metacarpals
(palm)

5   4   3   2   1

Metacarpal Bones

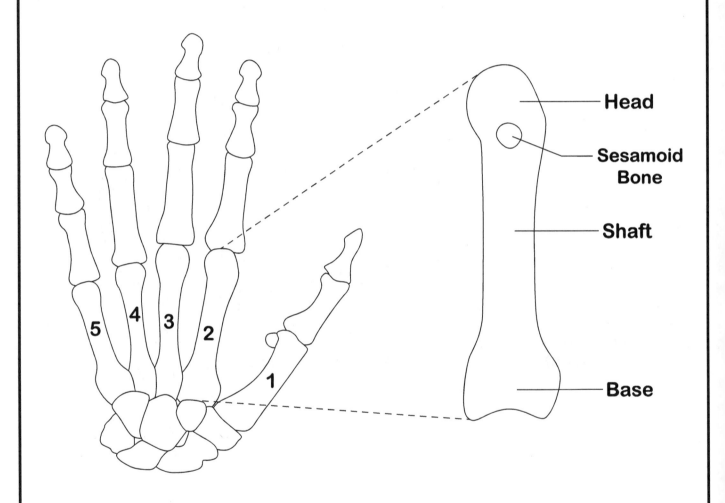

Phalanges of The Hand

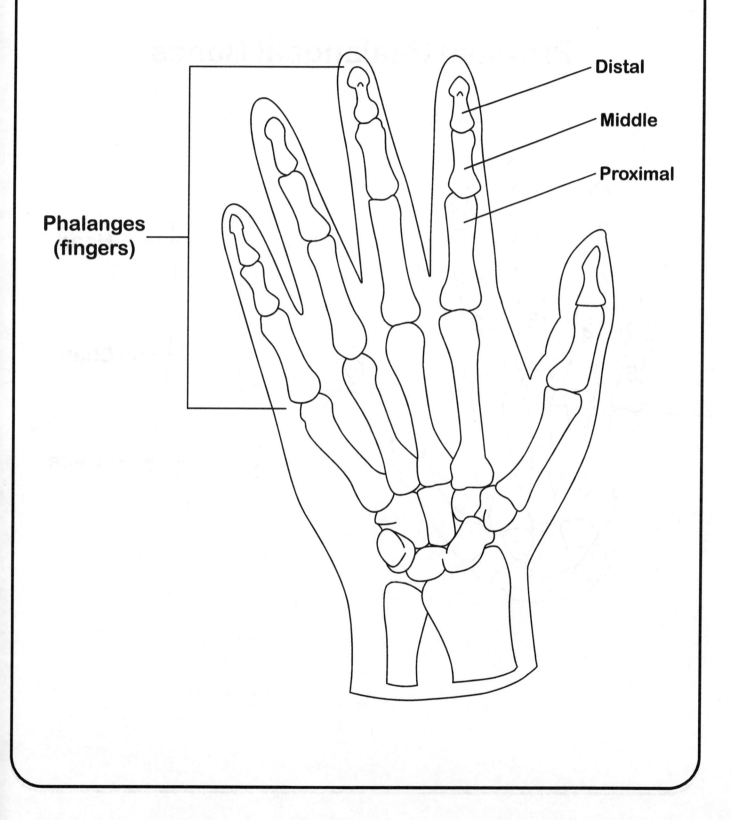

Distal

Middle

Proximal

Phalanges
(fingers)

Proximal Phalangeal Bones

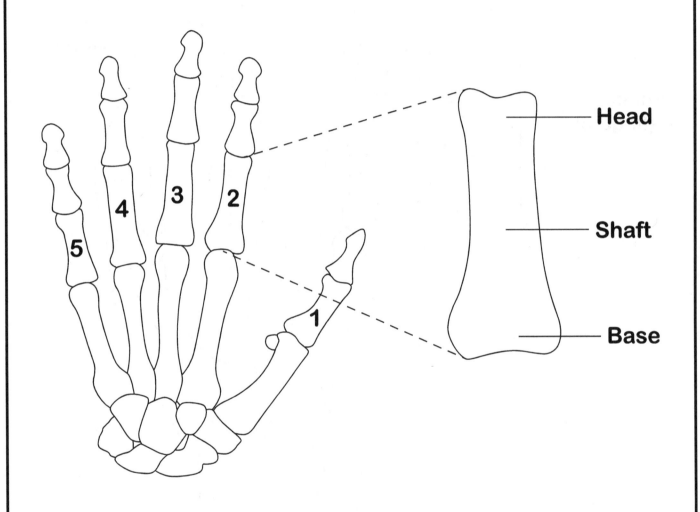

Middle Phalangeal Bones

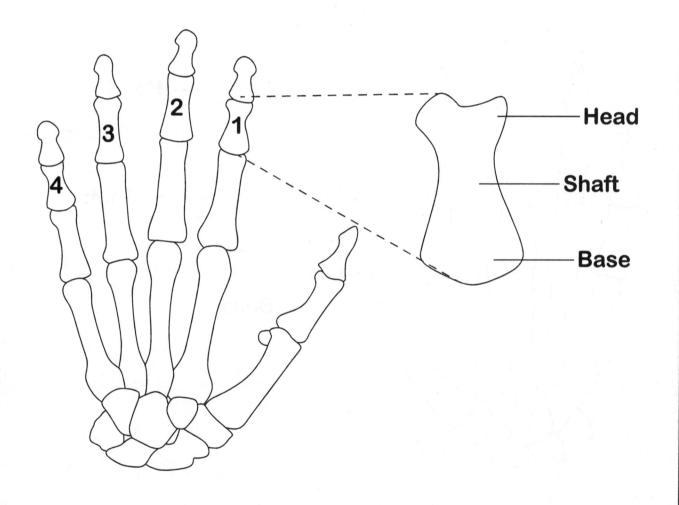

Distal Phalangeal Bones

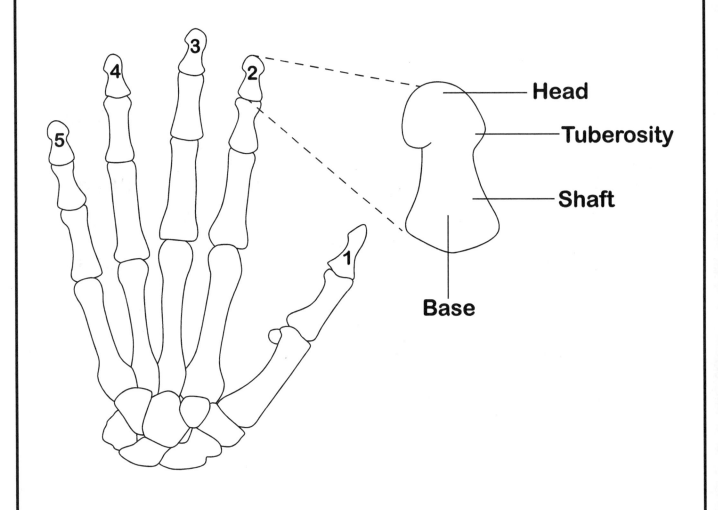

Head

Tuberosity

Shaft

Base

Metacarpal Bone And Phalanges
Of The Third Finger
Of The Right Hand

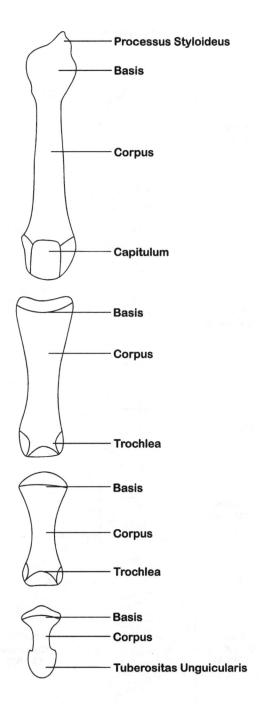

Processus Styloideus

Basis

Corpus

Capitulum

Basis

Corpus

Trochlea

Basis

Corpus

Trochlea

Basis

Corpus

Tuberositas Unguicularis

From The Dorsal Surface

Spine

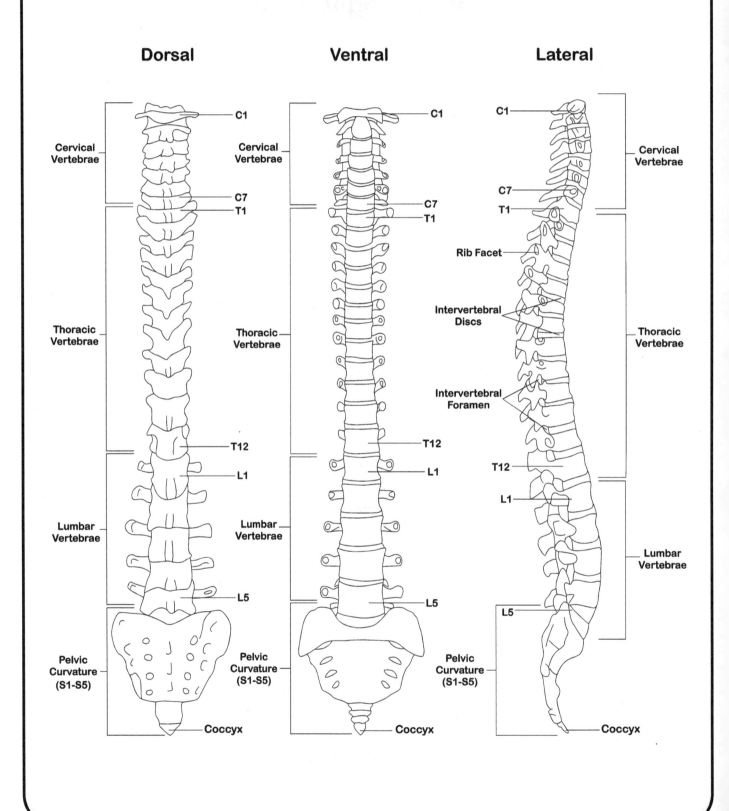

Dorsal

Cervical Vertebrae

C1

C7

Thoracic Vertebrae

T12

L1

Lumbar Vertebrae

L5

Pelvic Curvature (S1-S5)

Coccyx

Ventral

C1

Cervical Vertebrae

C7

T1

Thoracic Vertebrae

T12

L1

Lumbar Vertebrae

L5

Pelvic Curvature (S1-S5)

Coccyx

Lateral

C1

Cervical Vertebrae

C7

T1

Rib Facet

Intervertebral Discs

Intervertebral Foramen

Thoracic Vertebrae

T12

L1

Lumbar Vertebrae

L5

Pelvic Curvature (S1-S5)

Coccyx

Sacrum

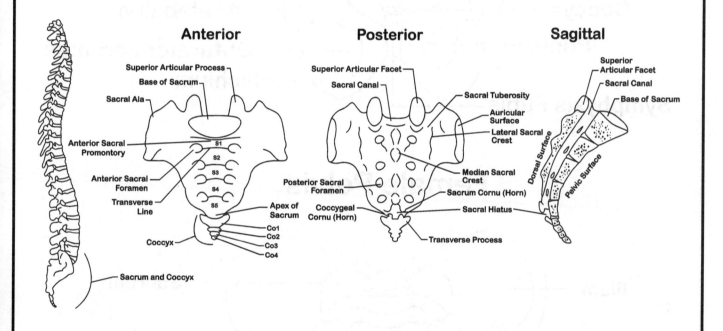

Anterior

- Superior Articular Process
- Base of Sacrum
- Sacral Ala
- Anterior Sacral Promontory
- Anterior Sacral Foramen
- Transverse Line
- S1
- S2
- S3
- S4
- S5
- Apex of Sacrum
- Coccyx
- Co1
- Co2
- Co3
- Co4
- Sacrum and Coccyx

Posterior

- Superior Articular Facet
- Sacral Canal
- Sacral Tuberosity
- Auricular Surface
- Lateral Sacral Crest
- Median Sacral Crest
- Posterior Sacral Foramen
- Sacrum Cornu (Horn)
- Coccygeal Cornu (Horn)
- Sacral Hiatus
- Transverse Process

Sagittal

- Superior Articular Facet
- Sacral Canal
- Base of Sacrum
- Dorsal Surface
- Pelvic Surface

Male Pelvis

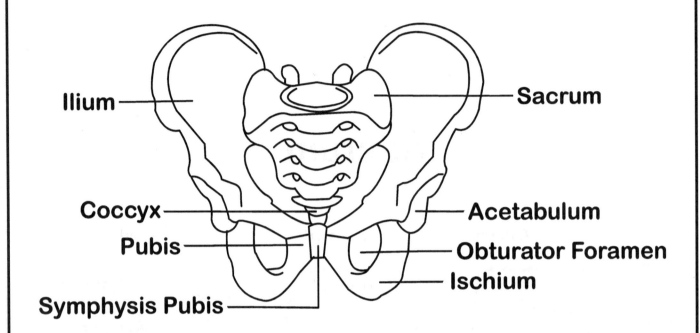

Ilium

Sacrum

Coccyx

Acetabulum

Pubis

Obturator Foramen

Ischium

Symphysis Pubis

Female Pelvis

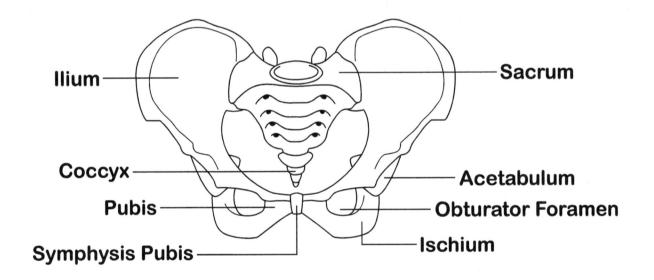

Ilium

Sacrum

Coccyx

Acetabulum

Pubis

Obturator Foramen

Symphysis Pubis

Ischium

Femur

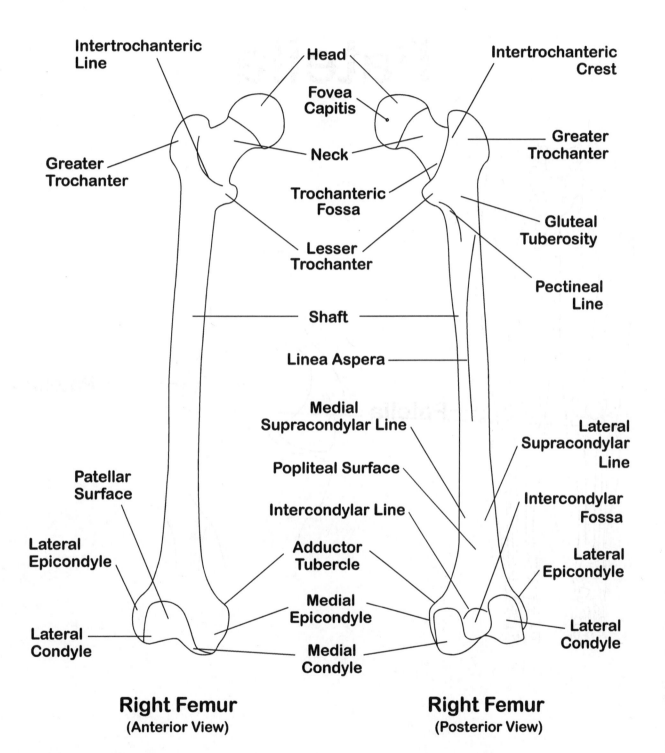

Intertrochanteric Line

Head

Fovea Capitis

Intertrochanteric Crest

Greater Trochanter

Neck

Greater Trochanter

Trochanteric Fossa

Gluteal Tuberosity

Lesser Trochanter

Pectineal Line

Shaft

Linea Aspera

Medial Supracondylar Line

Popliteal Surface

Lateral Supracondylar Line

Patellar Surface

Intercondylar Line

Intercondylar Fossa

Lateral Epicondyle

Adductor Tubercle

Lateral Epicondyle

Medial Epicondyle

Lateral Condyle

Lateral Condyle

Medial Condyle

Right Femur
(Anterior View)

Right Femur
(Posterior View)

Patella

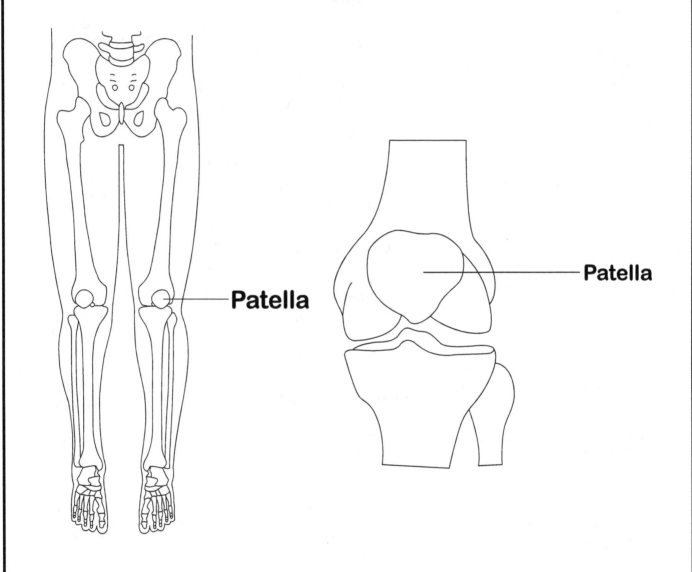

Patella

Patella

Patella

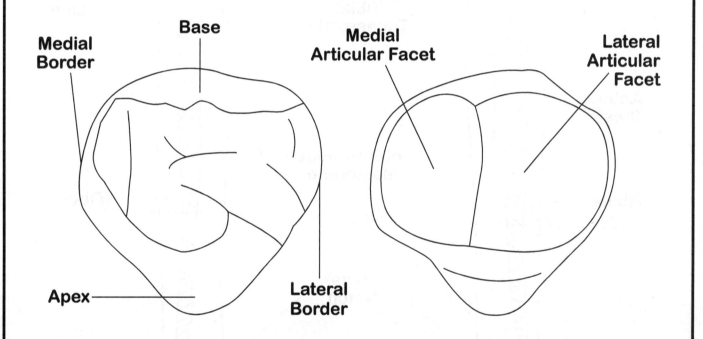

Medial Border

Base

Medial Articular Facet

Lateral Articular Facet

Apex

Lateral Border

(Anterior View)

(Posterior View)

Tibia

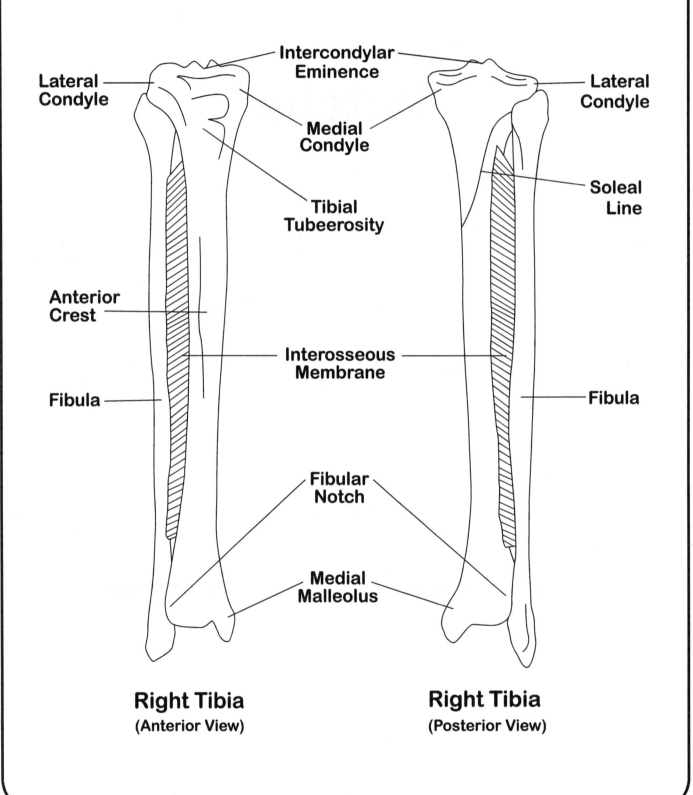

Intercondylar Eminence

Lateral Condyle

Lateral Condyle

Medial Condyle

Soleal Line

Tibial Tubeerosity

Anterior Crest

Interosseous Membrane

Fibula

Fibula

Fibular Notch

Medial Malleolus

Right Tibia
(Anterior View)

Right Tibia
(Posterior View)

Fibula

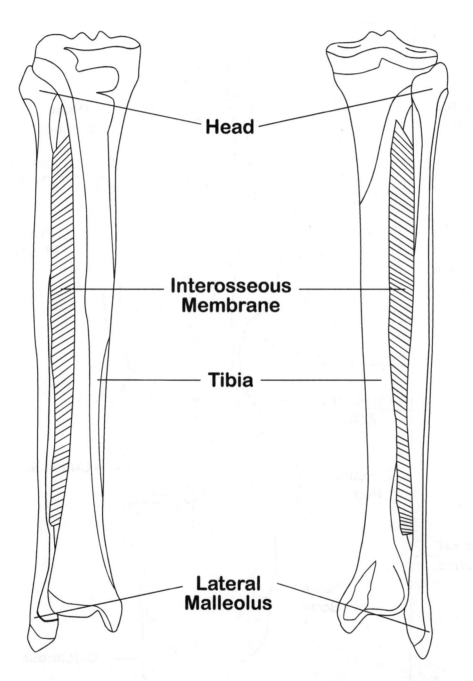

Head

Interosseous
Membrane

Tibia

Lateral
Malleolus

Right Fibula
(Anterior View)

Right Fibula
(Posterior View)

Foot Bones

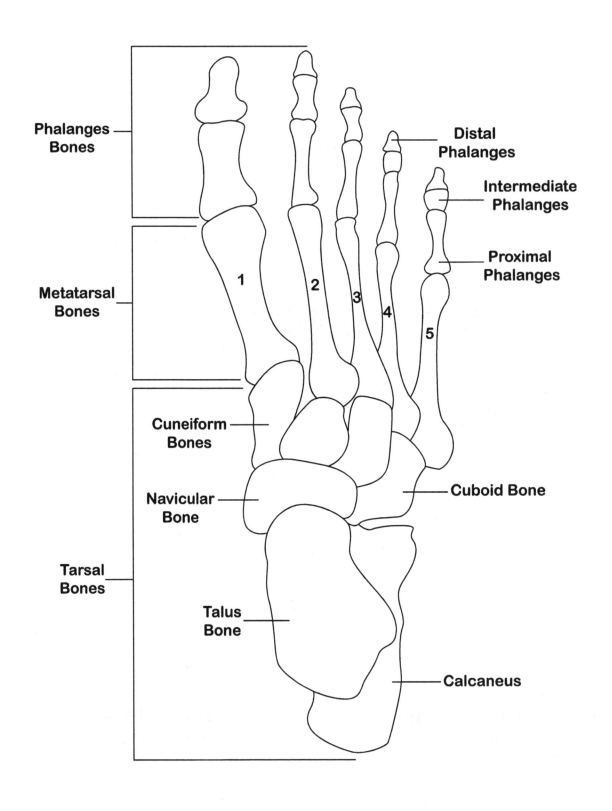

Phalanges Bones

Metatarsal Bones

Tarsal Bones

Distal Phalanges

Intermediate Phalanges

Proximal Phalanges

Cuneiform Bones

Navicular Bone

Cuboid Bone

Talus Bone

Calcaneus

1 2 3 4 5

Tarsal Bones

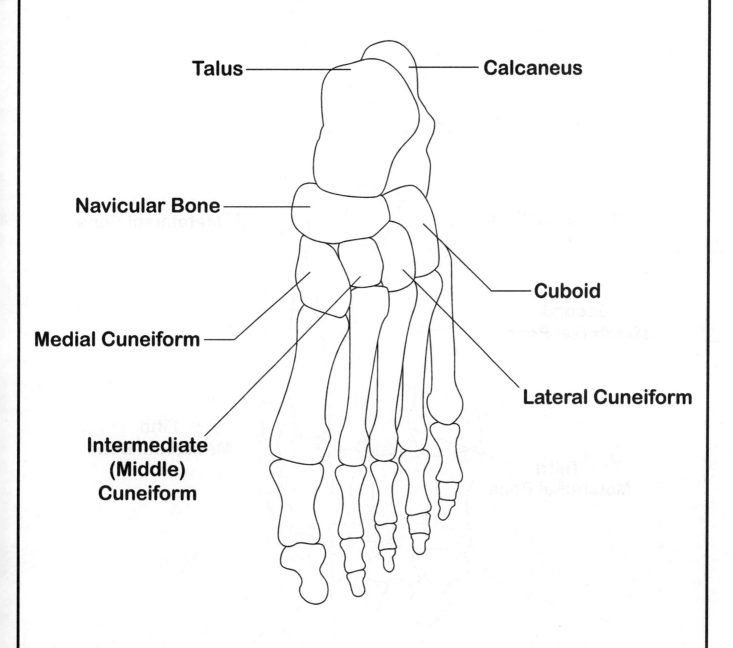

Talus

Calcaneus

Navicular Bone

Cuboid

Medial Cuneiform

Lateral Cuneiform

Intermediate
(Middle)
Cuneiform

Metatarsal Bones

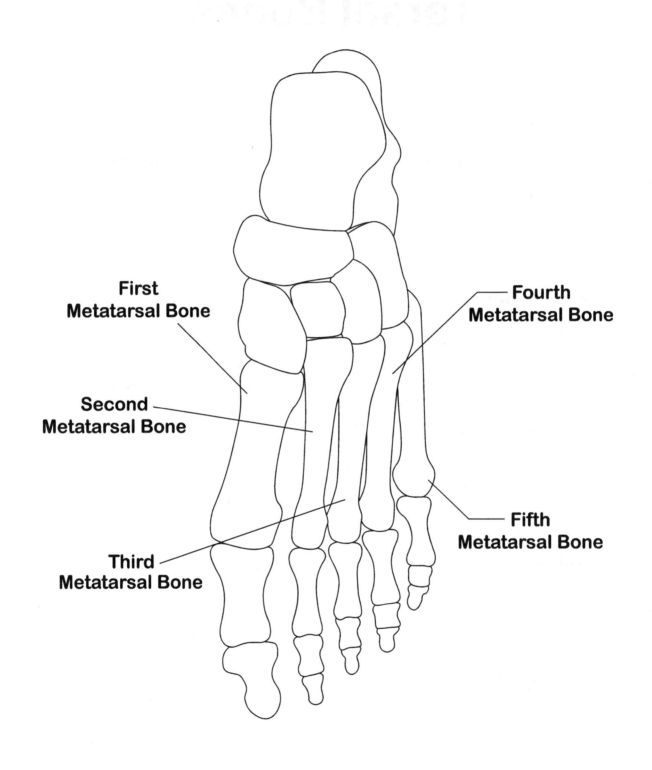

First Metatarsal Bone

Second Metatarsal Bone

Third Metatarsal Bone

Fourth Metatarsal Bone

Fifth Metatarsal Bone

Parts of Metatarsal Bones

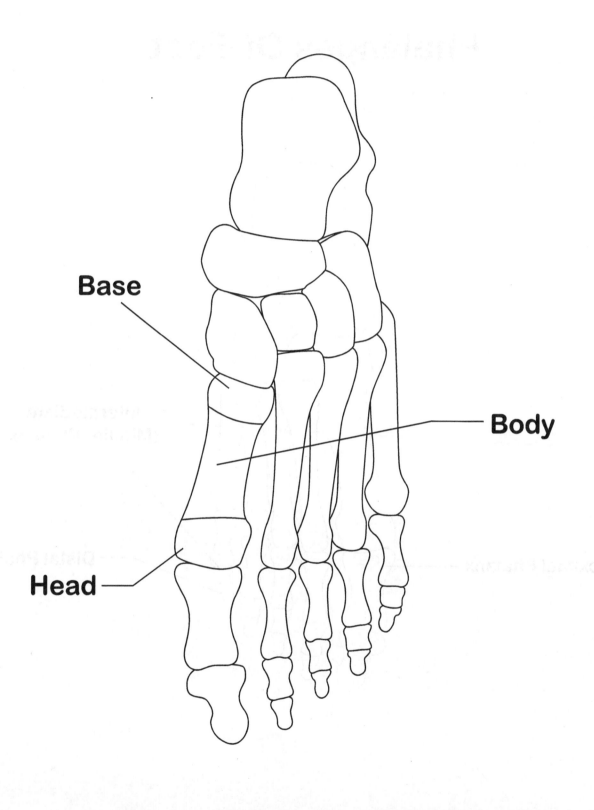

Phalanges Of Foot

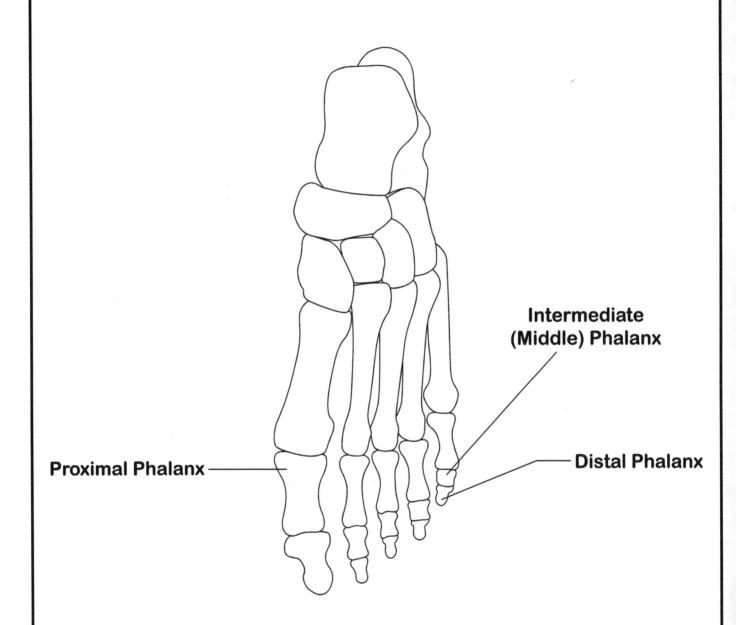

Intermediate (Middle) Phalanx

Distal Phalanx

Proximal Phalanx

Phalanges Of Foot
(Parts)

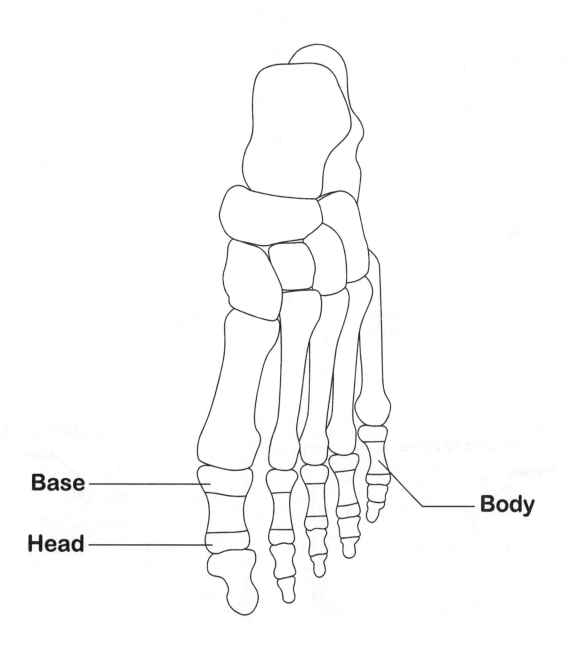

Base

Head

Body

Types Of Bones

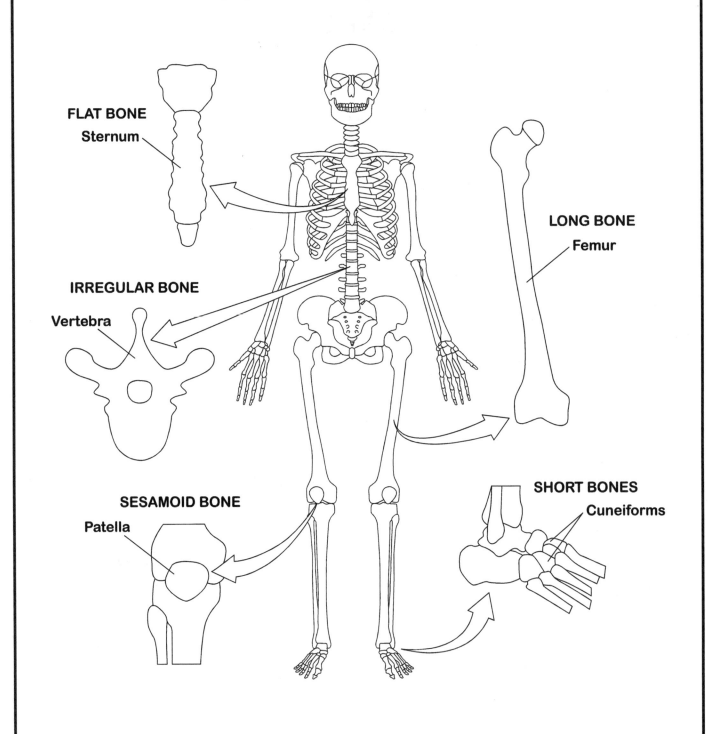

FLAT BONE
Sternum

LONG BONE
Femur

IRREGULAR BONE
Vertebra

SESAMOID BONE
Patella

SHORT BONES
Cuneiforms

Types of Bone Fractures

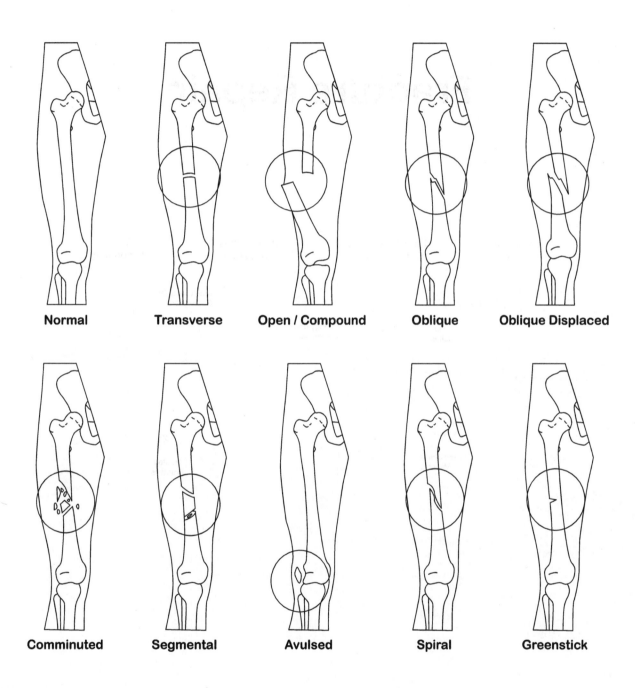

Normal   Transverse   Open / Compound   Oblique   Oblique Displaced

Comminuted   Segmental   Avulsed   Spiral   Greenstick

Fracture Repair

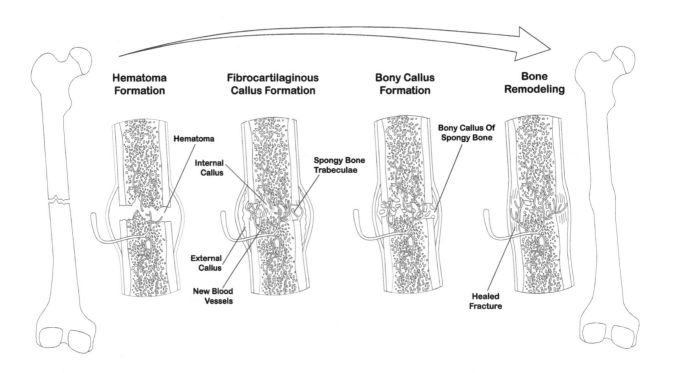

Hematoma Formation

Fibrocartilaginous Callus Formation

Bony Callus Formation

Bone Remodeling

Hematoma

Internal Callus

Spongy Bone Trabeculae

External Callus

New Blood Vessels

Bony Callus Of Spongy Bone

Healed Fracture

Bone Structure

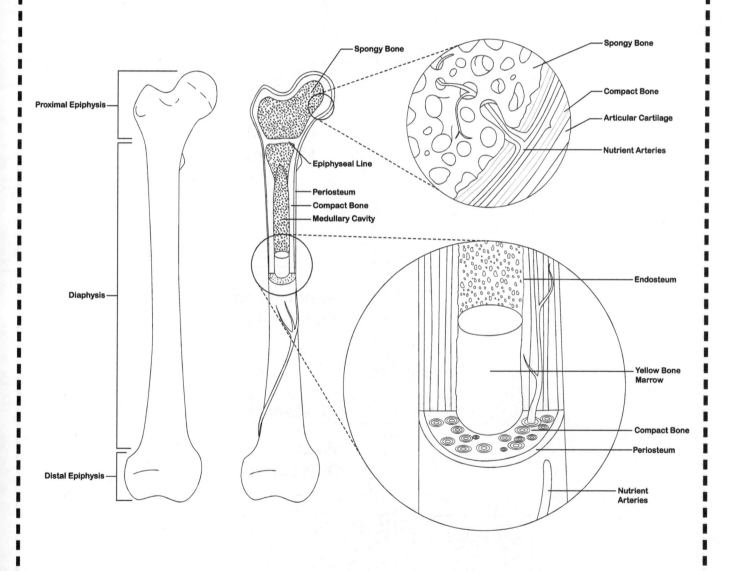

Proximal Epiphysis

Diaphysis

Distal Epiphysis

Spongy Bone

Epiphyseal Line

Periosteum

Compact Bone

Medullary Cavity

Spongy Bone

Compact Bone

Articular Cartilage

Nutrient Arteries

Endosteum

Yellow Bone Marrow

Compact Bone

Periosteum

Nutrient Arteries

Evolution
Of Bone Cells

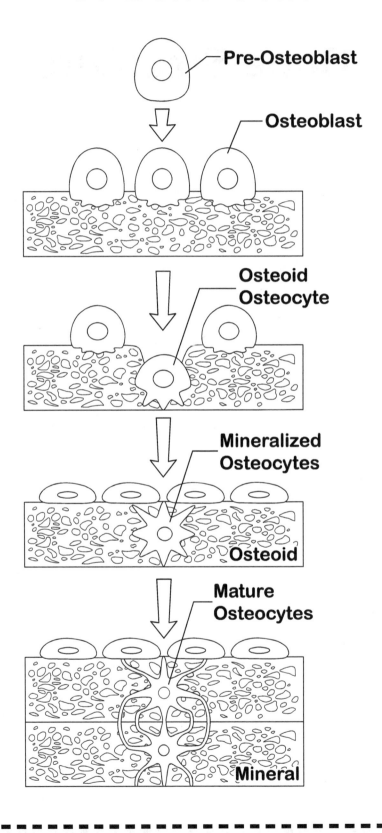

Bone Cross Section

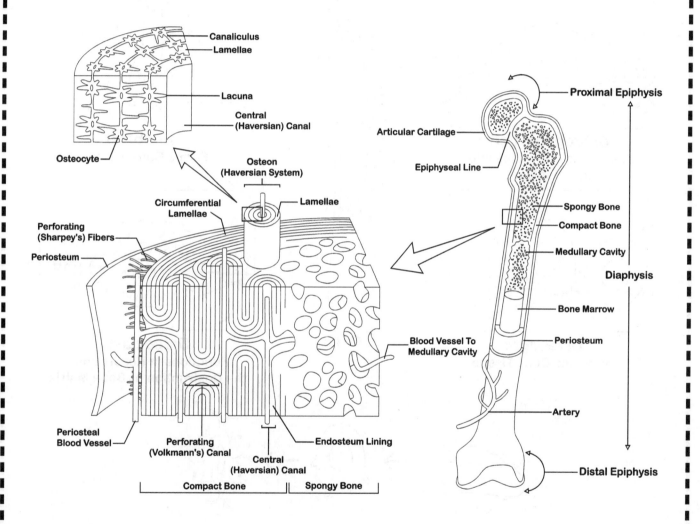

Canaliculus
Lamellae
Lacuna
Central (Haversian) Canal
Osteocyte
Osteon (Haversian System)
Circumferential Lamellae
Lamellae
Perforating (Sharpey's) Fibers
Periosteum
Periosteal Blood Vessel
Perforating (Volkmann's) Canal
Central (Haversian) Canal
Endosteum Lining
Blood Vessel To Medullary Cavity
Compact Bone
Spongy Bone

Proximal Epiphysis
Articular Cartilage
Epiphyseal Line
Spongy Bone
Compact Bone
Medullary Cavity
Diaphysis
Bone Marrow
Periosteum
Artery
Distal Epiphysis

Bone Cell Types

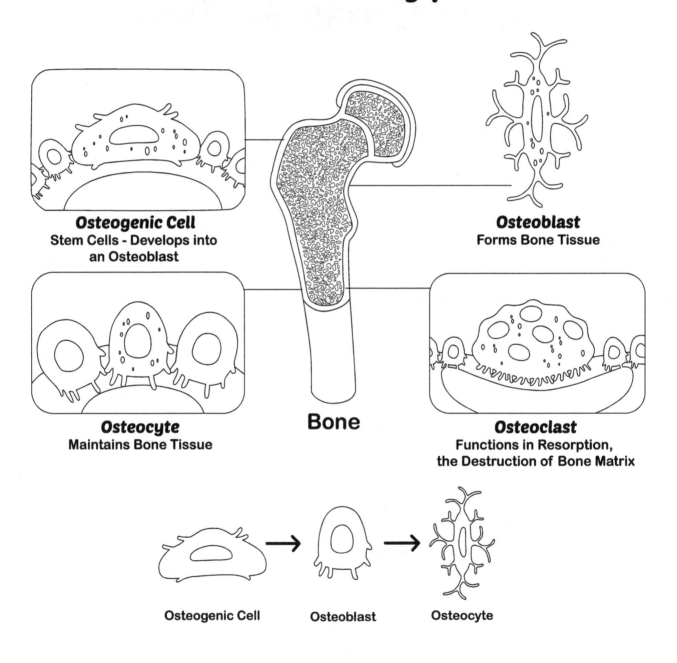

Osteogenic Cell
Stem Cells - Develops into
an Osteoblast

Osteoblast
Forms Bone Tissue

Osteocyte
Maintains Bone Tissue

Bone

Osteoclast
Functions in Resorption,
the Destruction of Bone Matrix

Osteogenic Cell → Osteoblast → Osteocyte

Spongy Bone and Compact Bone

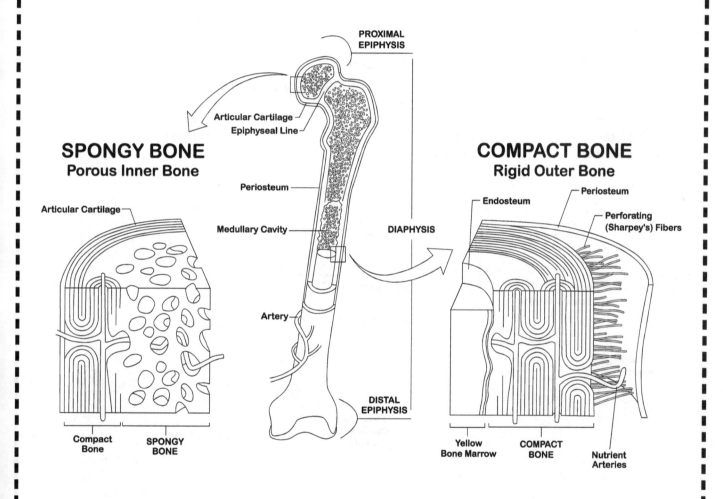

SPONGY BONE
Porous Inner Bone

COMPACT BONE
Rigid Outer Bone

PROXIMAL EPIPHYSIS

Articular Cartilage
Epiphyseal Line

Periosteum

Medullary Cavity

DIAPHYSIS

Artery

DISTAL EPIPHYSIS

Articular Cartilage

Compact Bone

SPONGY BONE

Endosteum

Periosteum

Perforating (Sharpey's) Fibers

Yellow Bone Marrow

COMPACT BONE

Nutrient Arteries

Growing Bones

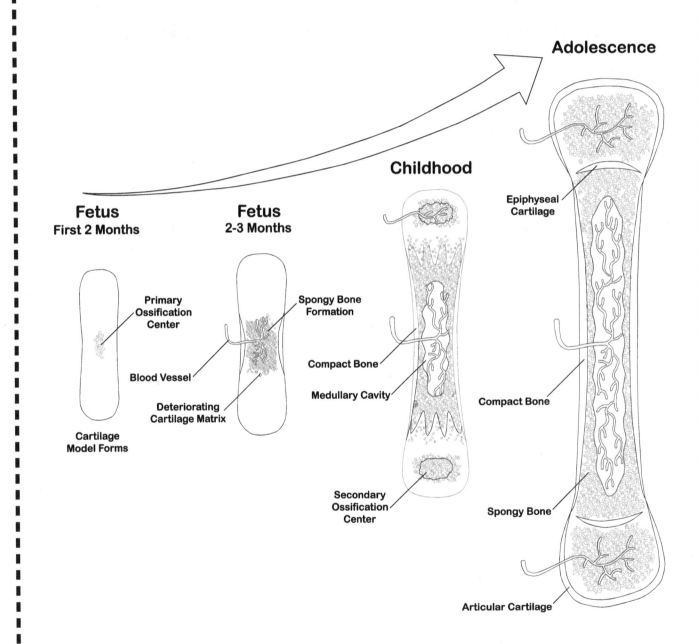

Adolescence

Childhood

Fetus
First 2 Months

Fetus
2-3 Months

Primary
Ossification
Center

Blood Vessel

Cartilage
Model Forms

Spongy Bone
Formation

Deteriorating
Cartilage Matrix

Compact Bone

Medullary Cavity

Secondary
Ossification
Center

Epiphyseal
Cartilage

Compact Bone

Spongy Bone

Articular Cartilage

Bone Healing

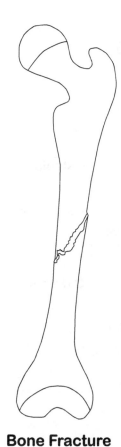

Bone Fracture

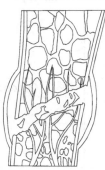

Hematoma

Inflammatory
Stage

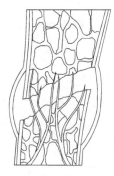

Soft Callus

Blood Vessels
Formation

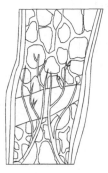

Hard Callus

Healed
Fracture

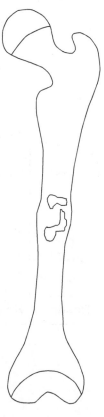

Bone Remodeling

Bone Remodelling Process

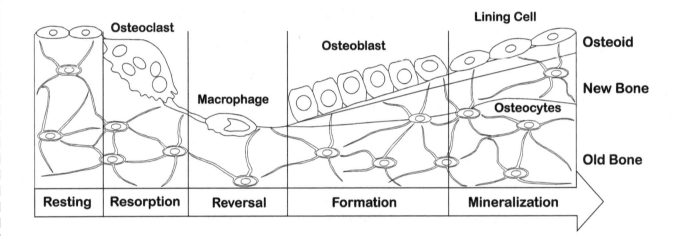

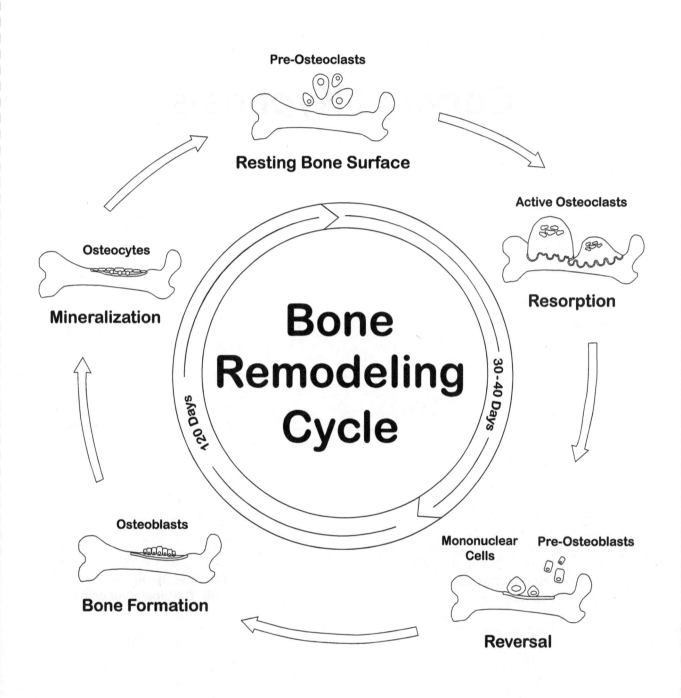

Cervical Kyphosis

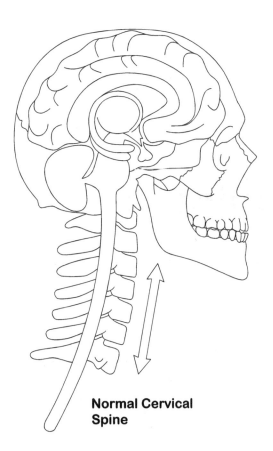

**Normal Cervical
Spine**

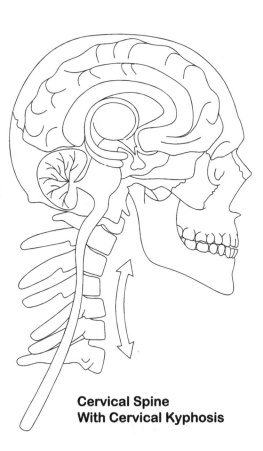

**Cervical Spine
With Cervical Kyphosis**

Cervical Spondylosis

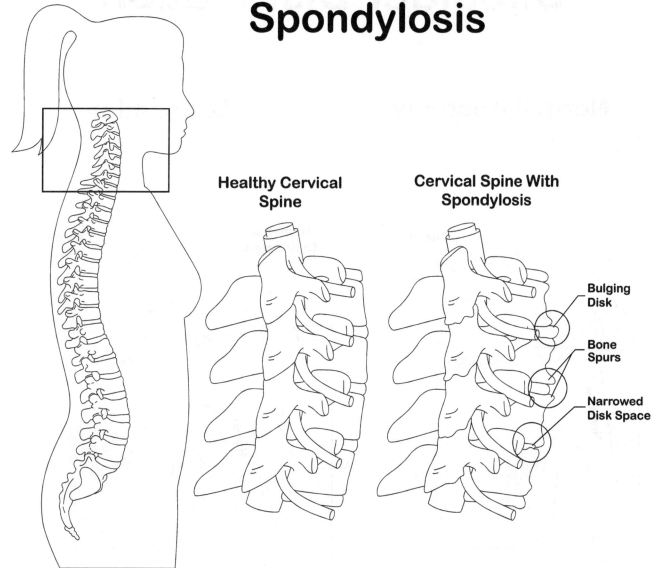

Healthy Cervical Spine

Cervical Spine With Spondylosis

Bulging Disk

Bone Spurs

Narrowed Disk Space

Shoulder Dislocation

Normal Anatomy

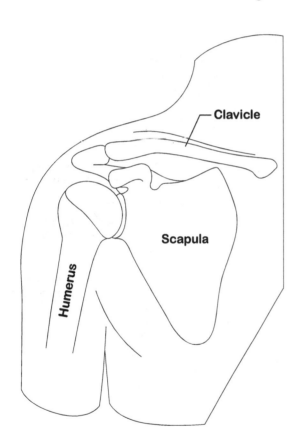

Clavicle

Scapula

Humerus

Dislocation

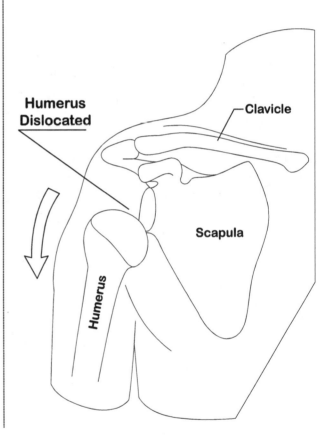

Humerus
Dislocated

Clavicle

Scapula

Humerus

Three Types Of Shoulder Dislocation

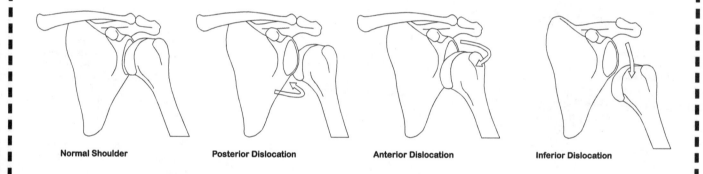

Normal Shoulder   Posterior Dislocation   Anterior Dislocation   Inferior Dislocation

Osteoporosis

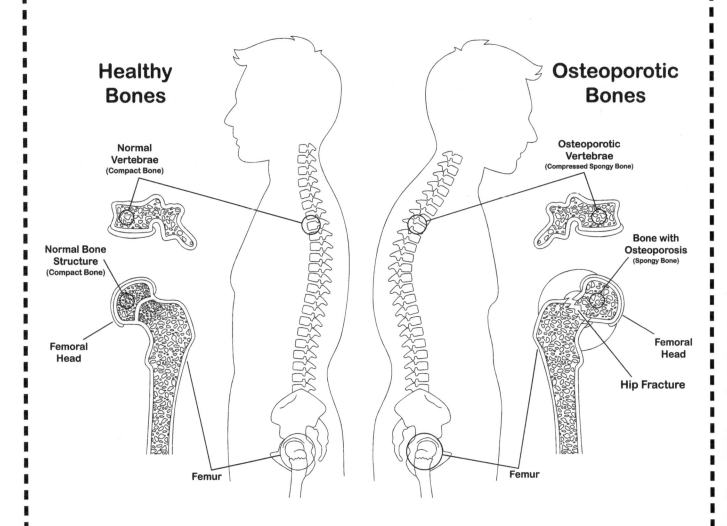

Healthy Bones

Normal Vertebrae (Compact Bone)

Normal Bone Structure (Compact Bone)

Femoral Head

Femur

Osteoporotic Bones

Osteoporotic Vertebrae (Compressed Spongy Bone)

Bone with Osteoporosis (Spongy Bone)

Femoral Head

Hip Fracture

Femur

Paget's Disease of Bone

Figure 1 - The Bones Commonly Affected By Paget's Disease

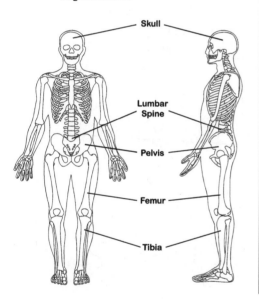

Skull

Lumbar Spine

Pelvis

Femur

Tibia

Figure 2 - Normal Bone Compared With Pagetic Bone

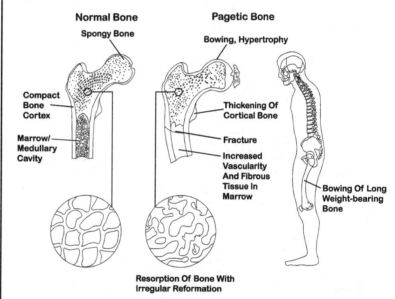

Normal Bone

Spongy Bone

Pagetic Bone

Bowing, Hypertrophy

Compact Bone Cortex

Marrow/ Medullary Cavity

Thickening Of Cortical Bone

Fracture

Increased Vascularity And Fibrous Tissue In Marrow

Bowing Of Long Weight-bearing Bone

Resorption Of Bone With Irregular Reformation

Scoliosis

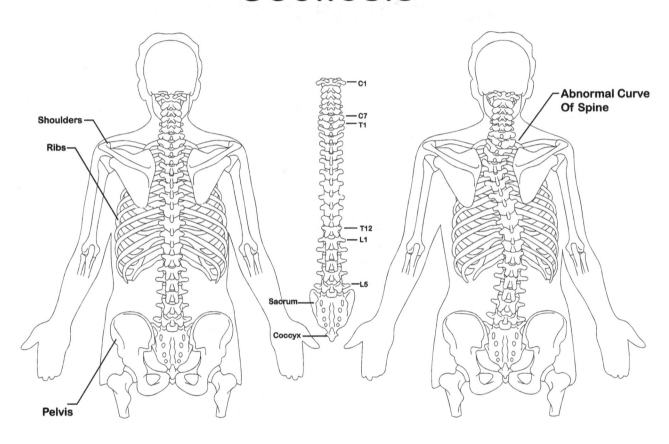

Shoulders

Ribs

Pelvis

C1

C7
T1

T12
L1

L5

Sacrum

Coccyx

Abnormal Curve
Of Spine

Healthy

Scoliosis

Types Of Scoliosis

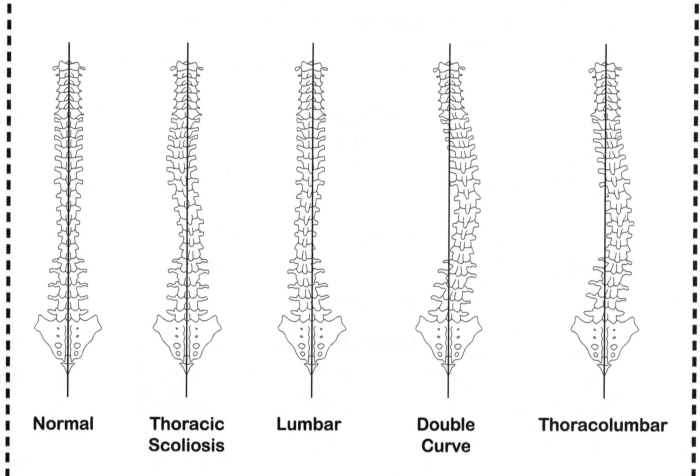

| Normal | Thoracic Scoliosis | Lumbar | Double Curve | Thoracolumbar |

Kyphosis

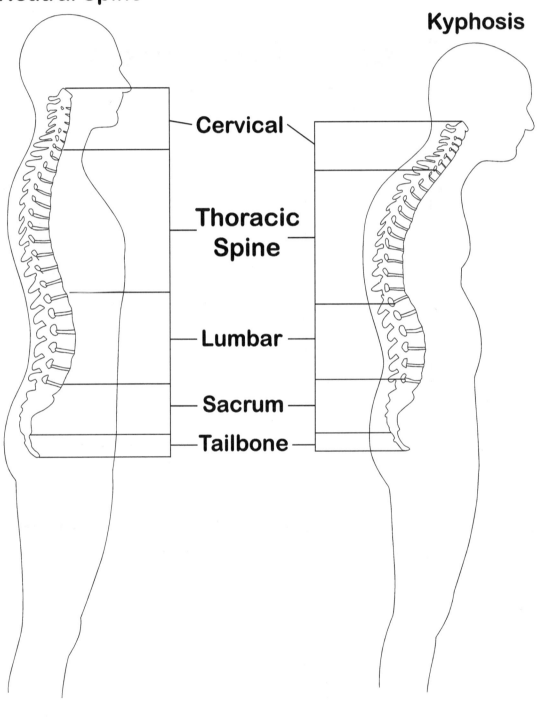

Neutral Spine

Kyphosis

Cervical

Thoracic
Spine

Lumbar

Sacrum

Tailbone

Lordosis

Normal

Lumbar Lordosis

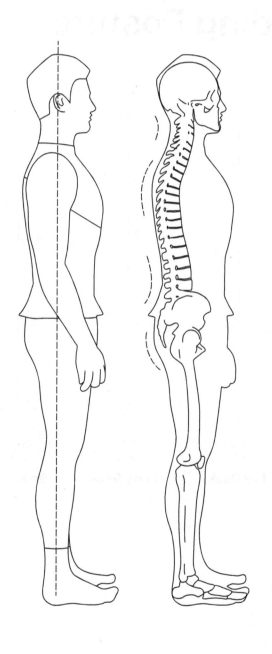

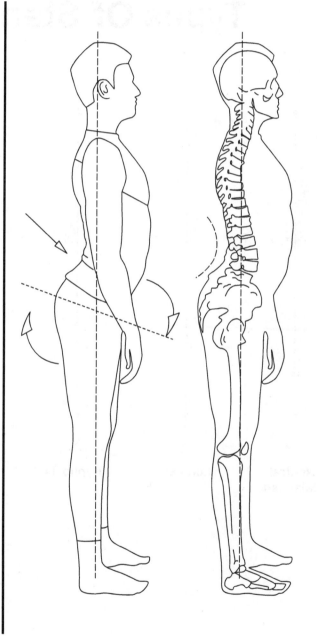

Types Of Standing Posture

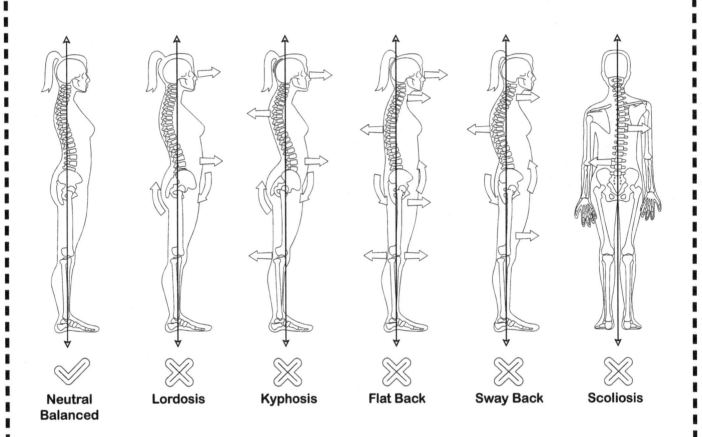

Neutral
Balanced

Lordosis

Kyphosis

Flat Back

Sway Back

Scoliosis

Spinal Deformity Types

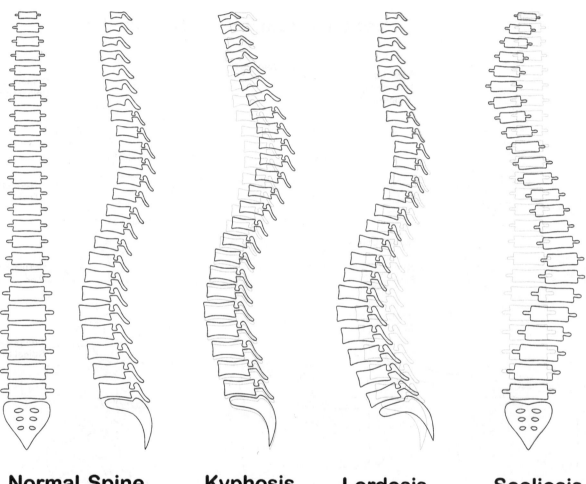

Normal Spine   **Kyphosis**   **Lordosis**   **Scoliosis**

Disc Herniation

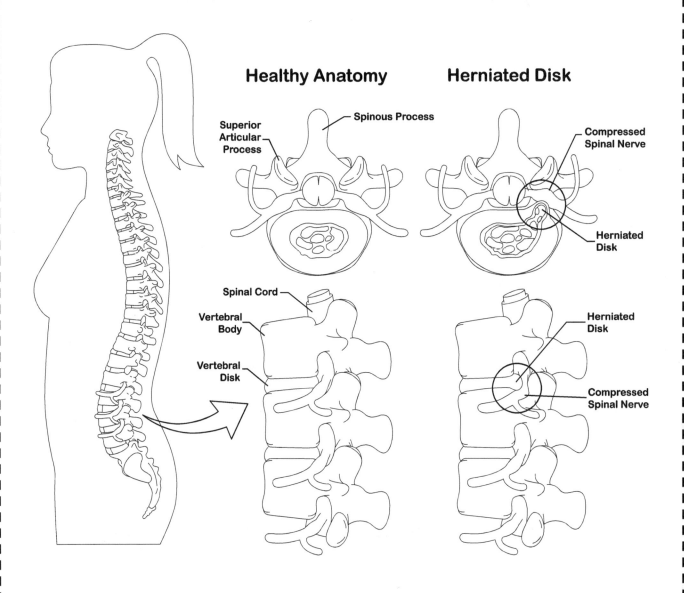

Healthy Anatomy

Herniated Disk

Spinous Process

Superior Articular Process

Compressed Spinal Nerve

Herniated Disk

Spinal Cord

Vertebral Body

Vertebral Disk

Herniated Disk

Compressed Spinal Nerve

Osteoarthritis Spine

Healthy Spine

Body Of Vertebra

Intervertebral Disk

Osteoarthritis Spine

Bone Spurring

Narrowed Disk

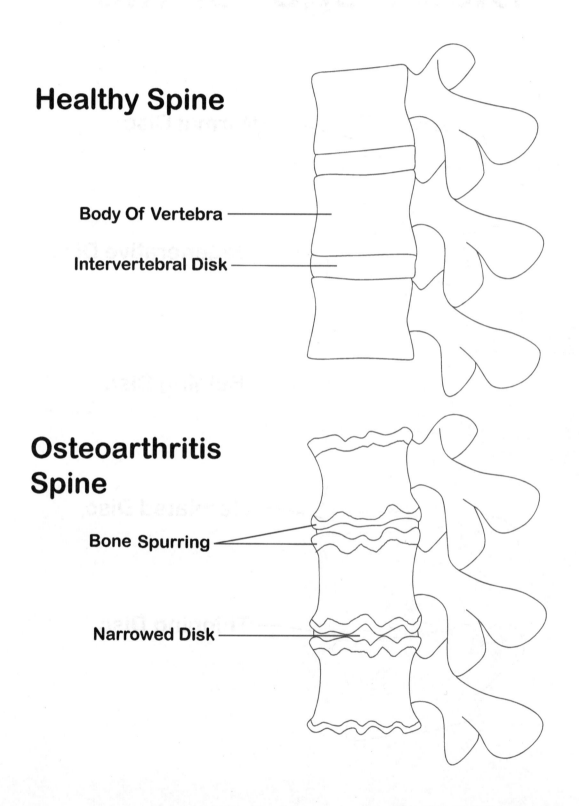

Disk Degeneration

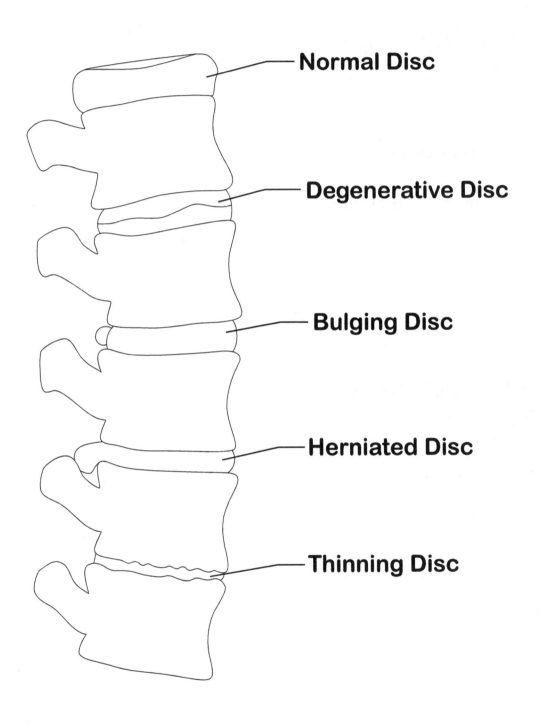

Normal Disc

Degenerative Disc

Bulging Disc

Herniated Disc

Thinning Disc

Kyphoplasty

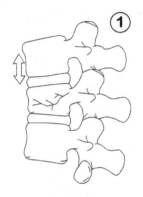

Compressed Vertebrae

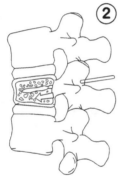

Balloon Is Inserted To The Compressed Vertebrae

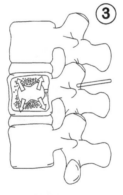

Balloon Inflated

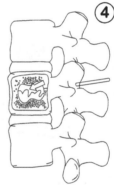

Balloon Removed And Cement Is Inserted

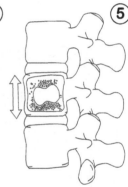

The Cement Hardens Restoring Vertebral Height

Rickets

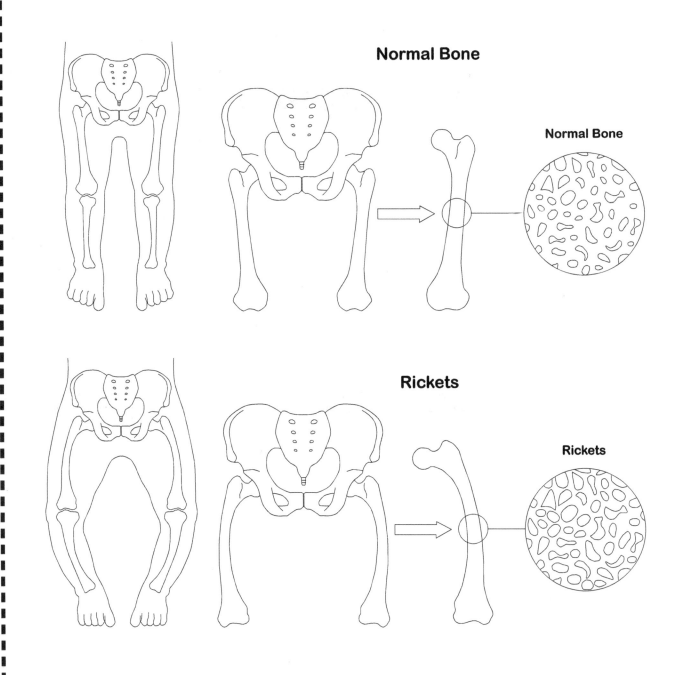

Normal Bone

Normal Bone

Rickets

Rickets

Hip Labral Tear

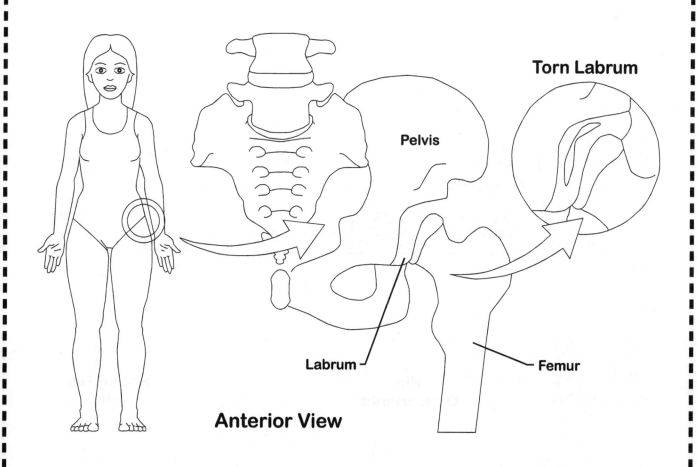

Torn Labrum

Pelvis

Labrum

Femur

Anterior View

Hip Osteoarthritis

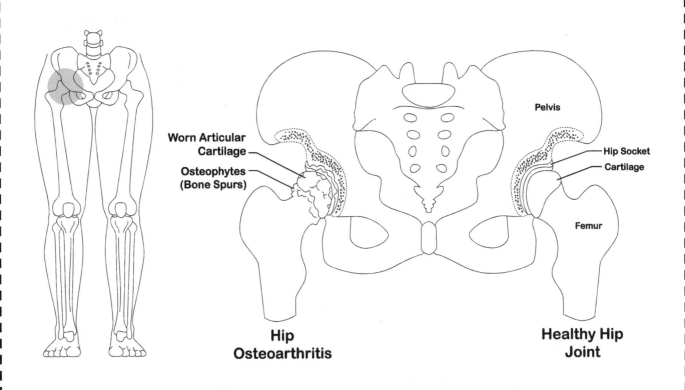

Worn Articular
Cartilage

Osteophytes
(Bone Spurs)

Pelvis

Hip Socket

Cartilage

Femur

Hip
Osteoarthritis

Healthy Hip
Joint

Total Hip Replacement

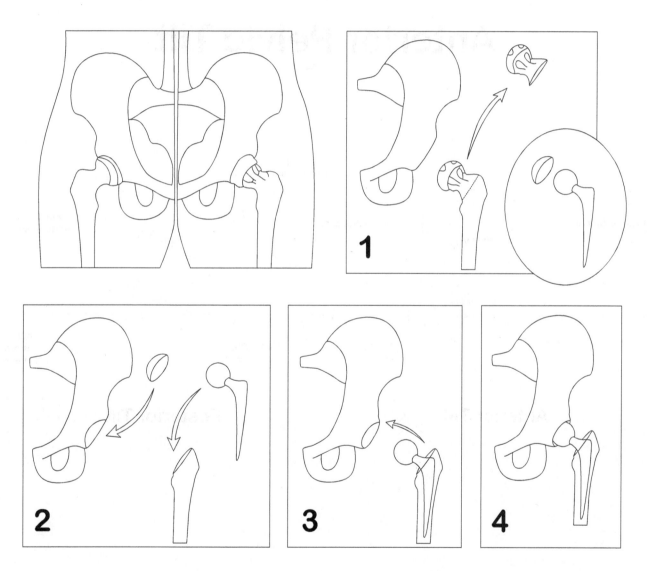

Anterior Pelvic Tilt

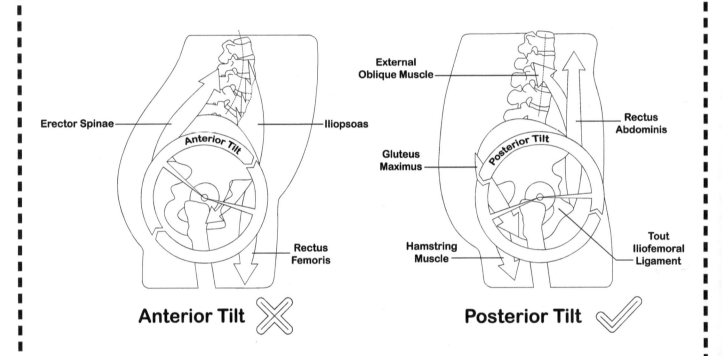

Erector Spinae

Iliopsoas

Anterior Tilt

Rectus Femoris

Anterior Tilt ✕

External Oblique Muscle

Gluteus Maximus

Posterior Tilt

Rectus Abdominis

Tout Iliofemoral Ligament

Hamstring Muscle

Posterior Tilt ✓

Leg Length Discrepancy

Normal Position Of Leg

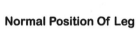

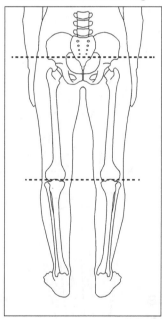

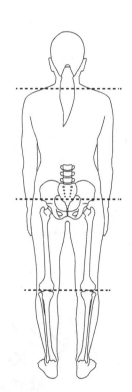

Leg Length Discrepancy

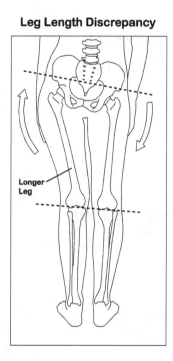

Longer
Leg

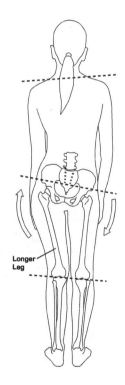

Longer
Leg

Mechanism Of ACL Injury

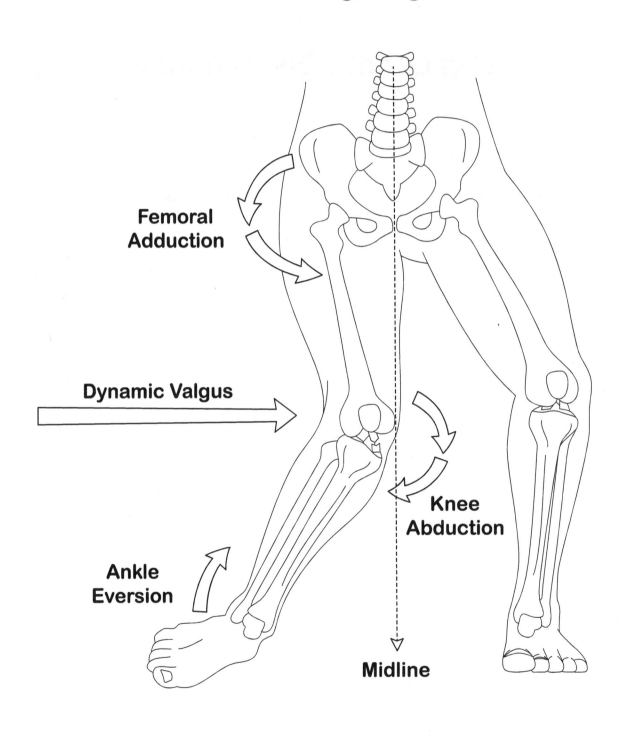

Femoral Adduction

Dynamic Valgus

Knee Abduction

Ankle Eversion

Midline

ACL Injury

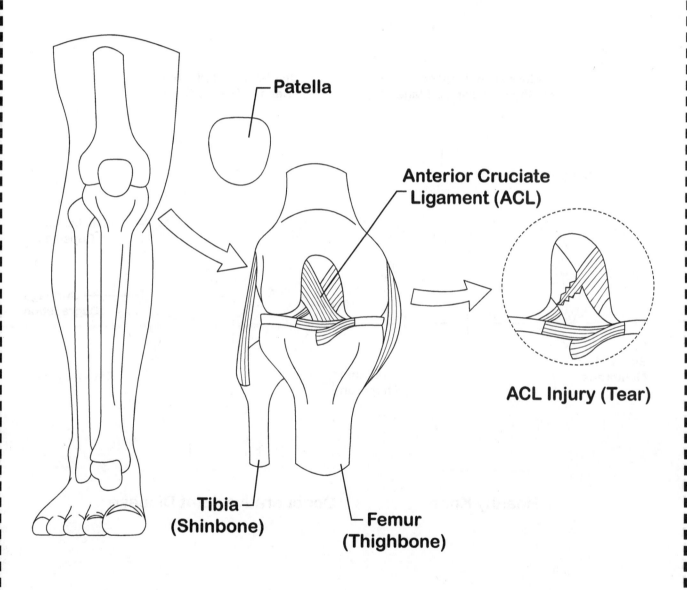

Patella

Anterior Cruciate
Ligament (ACL)

ACL Injury (Tear)

Tibia
(Shinbone)

Femur
(Thighbone)

Osteoarthritis

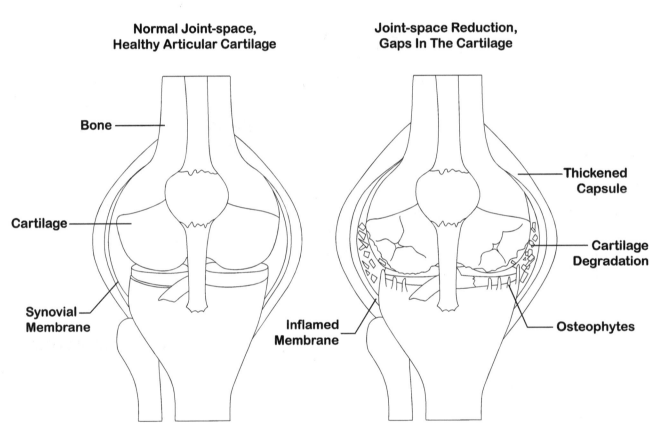

Normal Joint-space,
Healthy Articular Cartilage

Joint-space Reduction,
Gaps In The Cartilage

Bone

Cartilage

Synovial
Membrane

Thickened
Capsule

Cartilage
Degradation

Inflamed
Membrane

Osteophytes

Healthy Knee

Degenerative Joint Disease

Arthrosis

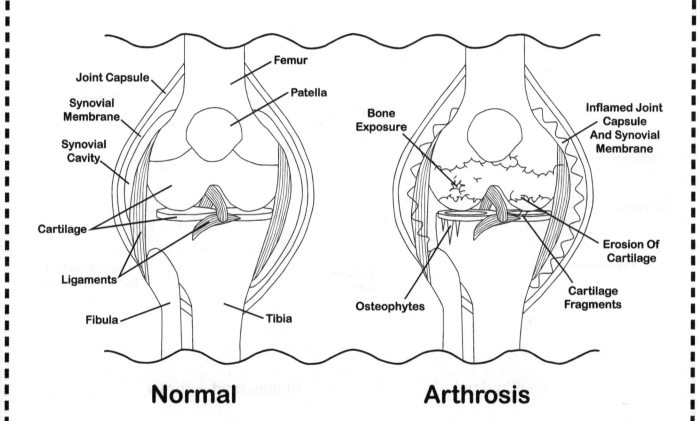

Normal

Joint Capsule
Synovial Membrane
Synovial Cavity
Cartilage
Ligaments
Fibula
Femur
Patella
Tibia

Arthrosis

Bone Exposure
Osteophytes
Inflamed Joint Capsule And Synovial Membrane
Erosion Of Cartilage
Cartilage Fragments

Rheumatoid Arthritis

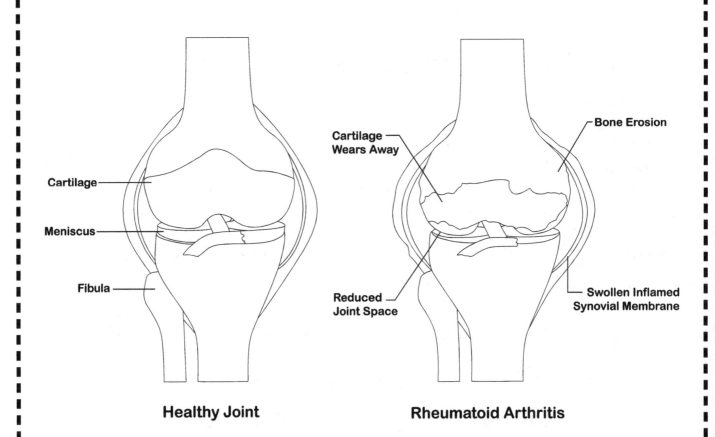

Cartilage

Meniscus

Fibula

Cartilage Wears Away

Reduced Joint Space

Bone Erosion

Swollen Inflamed Synovial Membrane

Healthy Joint

Rheumatoid Arthritis

Patellar Dislocation

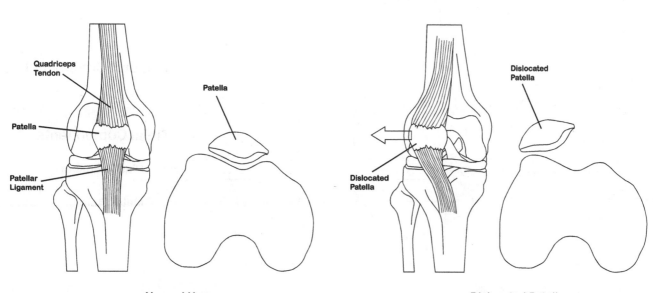

Normal Knee   Dislocated Patella

Total Knee Replacement

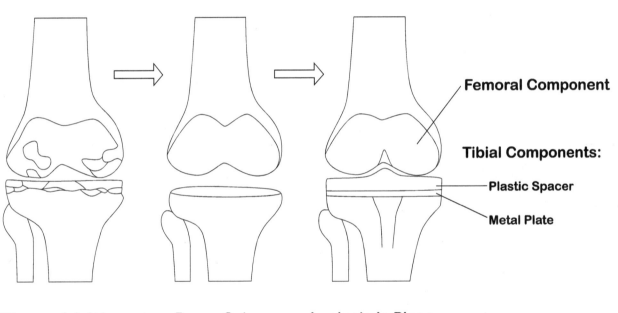

Femoral Component

Tibial Components:

Plastic Spacer

Metal Plate

Diseased Joint

**Bones Cut
And Shaped**

Implants In Place

Osteosarcoma

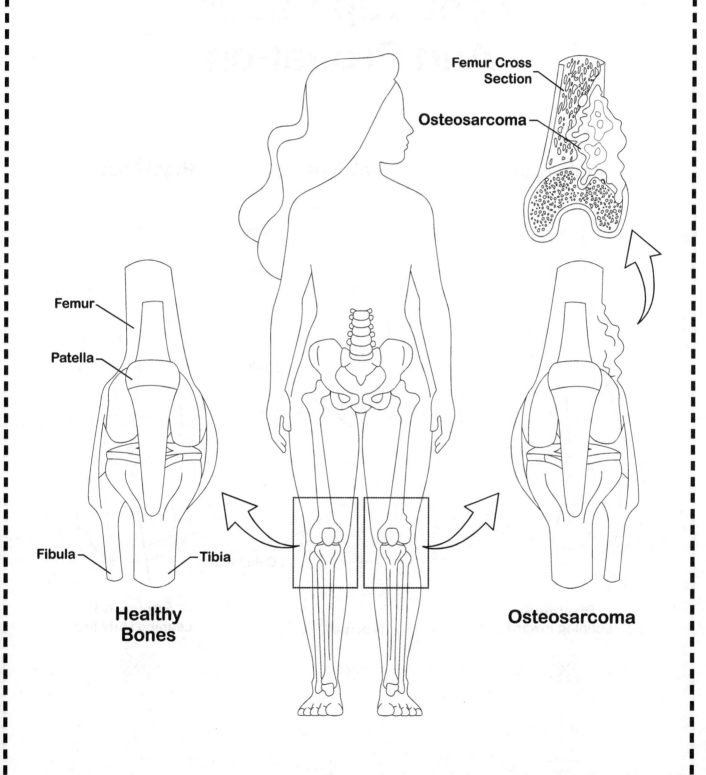

Foot Supination And Pronation

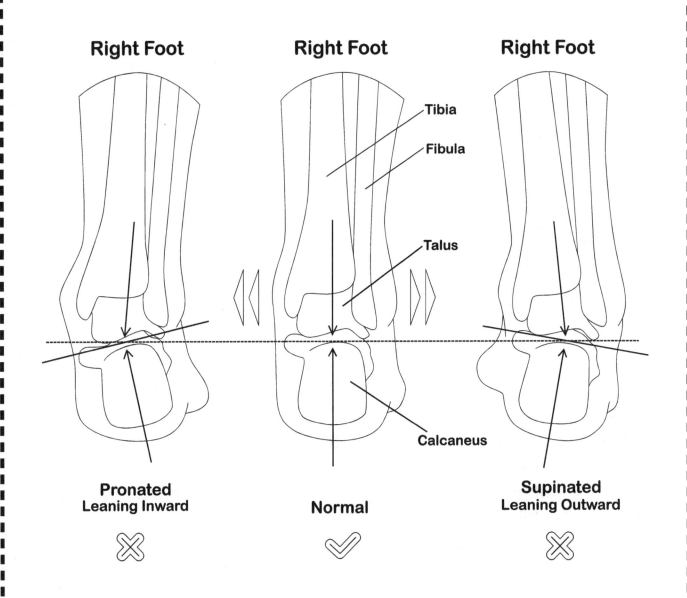

Right Foot **Right Foot** **Right Foot**

Tibia

Fibula

Talus

Calcaneus

Pronated
Leaning Inward

Normal

Supinated
Leaning Outward

Deformation Of The Foot

Flat Foot (Fallen Arch)			
Normal Foot			
Hollow Foot (High Arch)			

Foot Arch Deformities

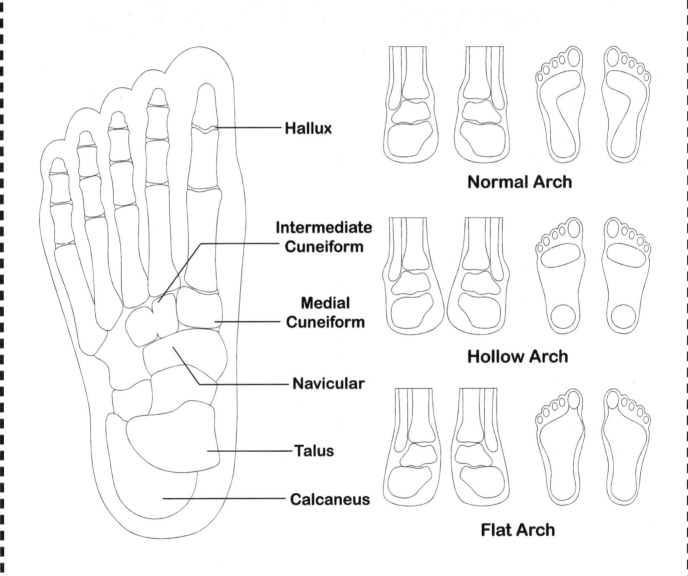

Hallux

Intermediate Cuneiform

Medial Cuneiform

Navicular

Talus

Calcaneus

Normal Arch

Hollow Arch

Flat Arch

Pathologies Of Foot

Normal Foot

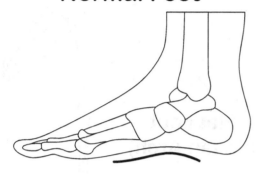 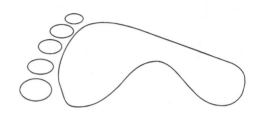

Flat Foot (Fallen Arch)

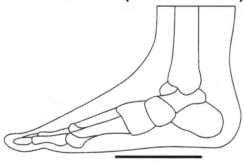 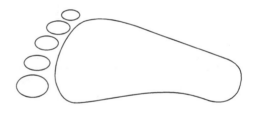

Hollow Foot (High Arch)

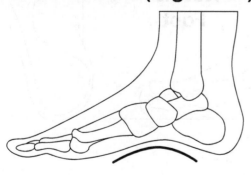 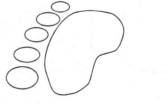

Flat Foot

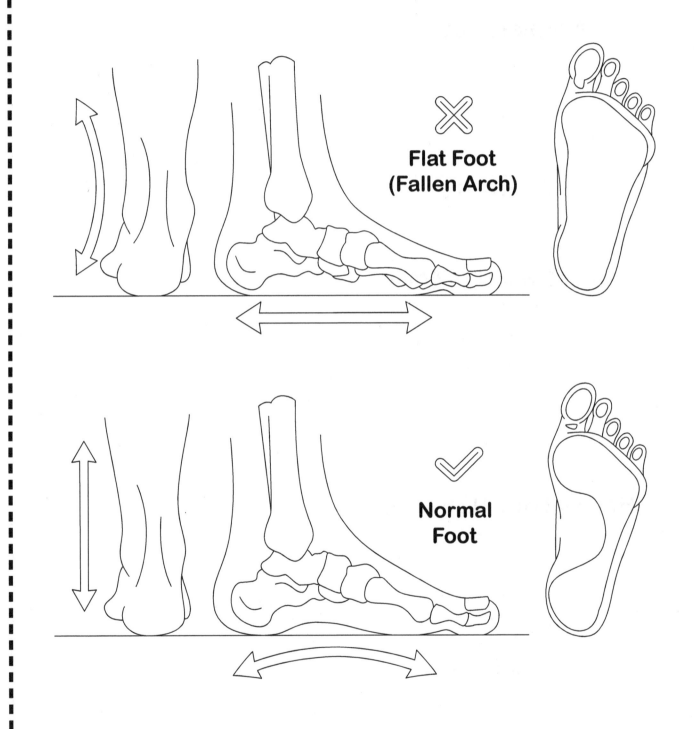

✗
**Flat Foot
(Fallen Arch)**

✓
**Normal
Foot**

Cavus Foot

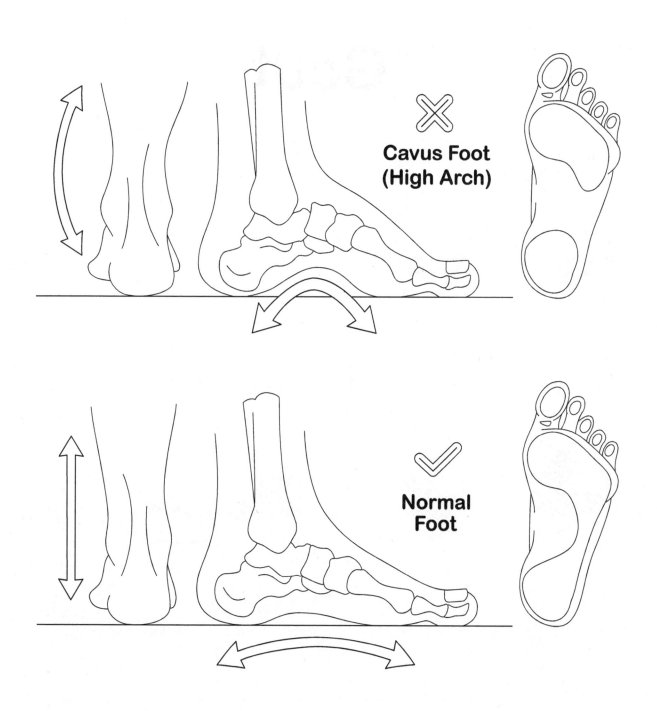

Cavus Foot
(High Arch)

Normal
Foot

Gout

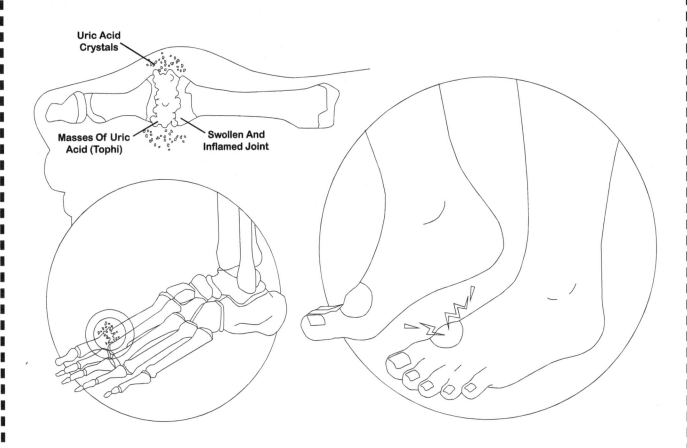

Uric Acid Crystals

Masses Of Uric Acid (Tophi)

Swollen And Inflamed Joint

Bunions

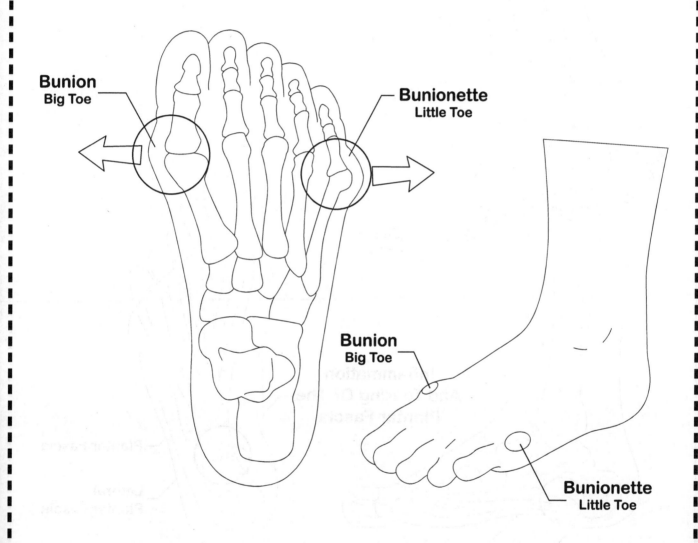

Bunion
Big Toe

Bunionette
Little Toe

Bunion
Big Toe

Bunionette
Little Toe

Plantar Fasciitis

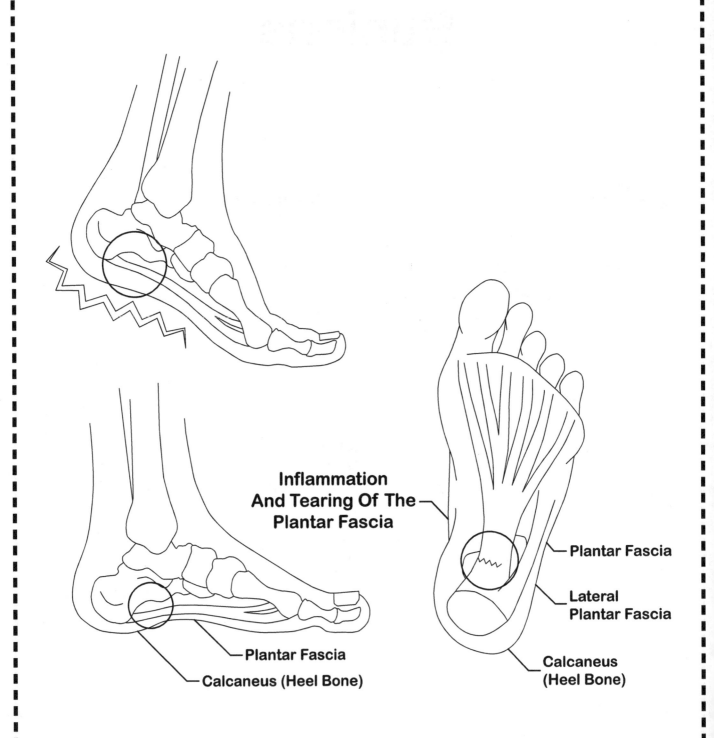

Inflammation
And Tearing Of The
Plantar Fascia

Plantar Fascia

Lateral
Plantar Fascia

Calcaneus
(Heel Bone)

Plantar Fascia

Calcaneus (Heel Bone)

Toe Deformities

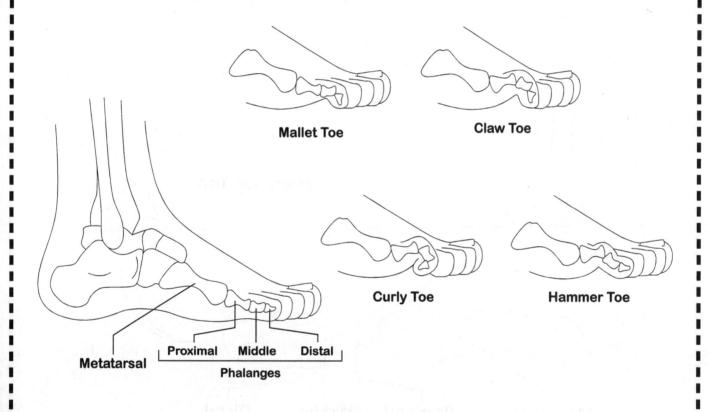

Mallet Toe

Claw Toe

Curly Toe

Hammer Toe

Metatarsal

Proximal Middle Distal
Phalanges

Hammer Toe

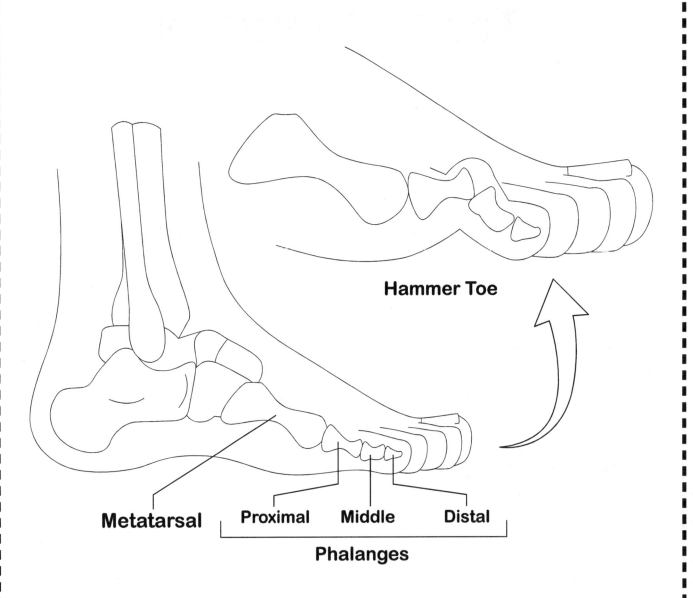

Hammer Toe

Metatarsal   **Proximal**   **Middle**   **Distal**

Phalanges

Finger Injury

Mallet Finger

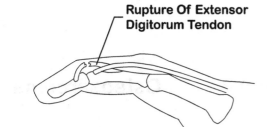

Rupture Of Extensor
Digitorum Tendon

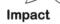

Impact

Jersey Finger

Rupture Of Flexor
Digitorum Profundus Tendon

Impact

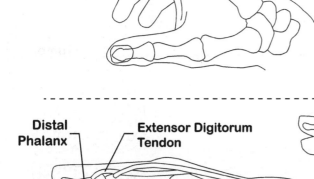

Distal
Phalanx

Extensor Digitorum
Tendon

Flexor Digitorum
Profundus Tendon

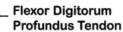

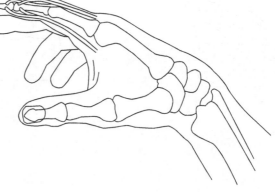

Bone Cancer

Chondrosarcoma

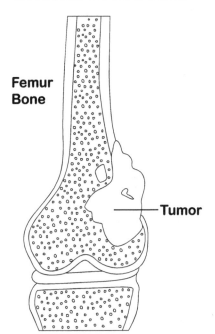

Femur
Bone

Tumor

Ewing's Sarcoma

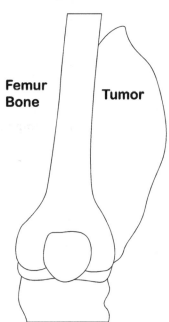

Femur
Bone

Tumor

Osteosarcoma

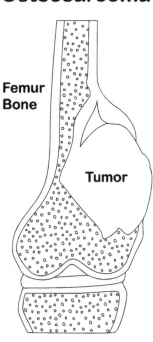

Femur
Bone

Tumor

Bone Tumor

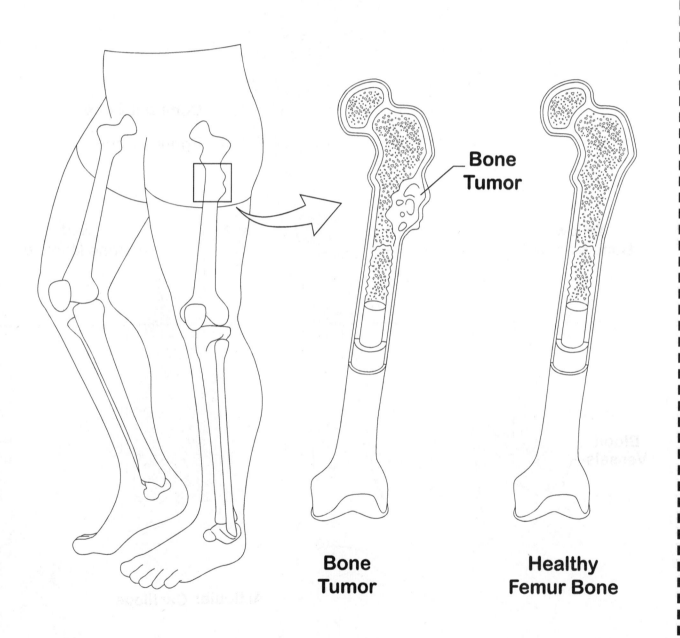

Bone
Tumor

Bone
Tumor

Healthy
Femur Bone

Bone Marrow

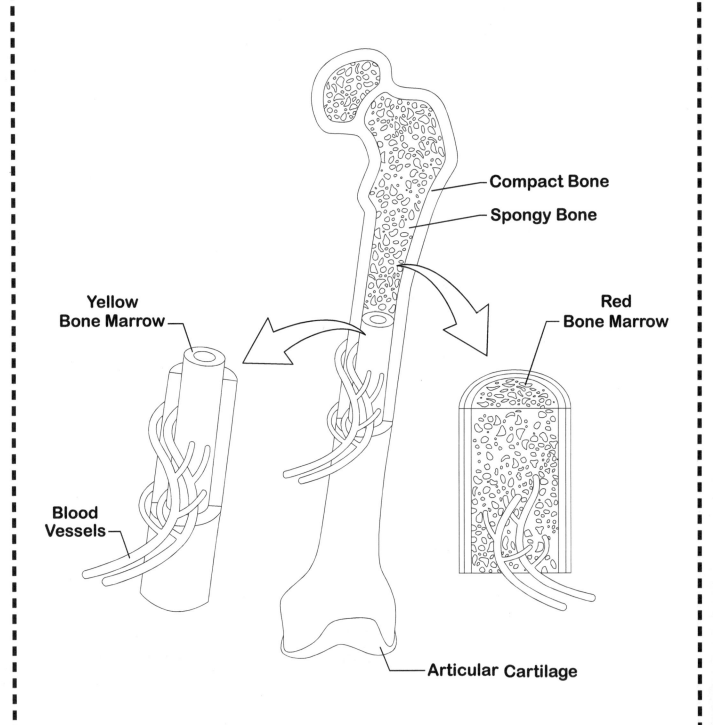

Compact Bone

Spongy Bone

Yellow
Bone Marrow

Red
Bone Marrow

Blood
Vessels

Articular Cartilage

Arthritis Joint Pain

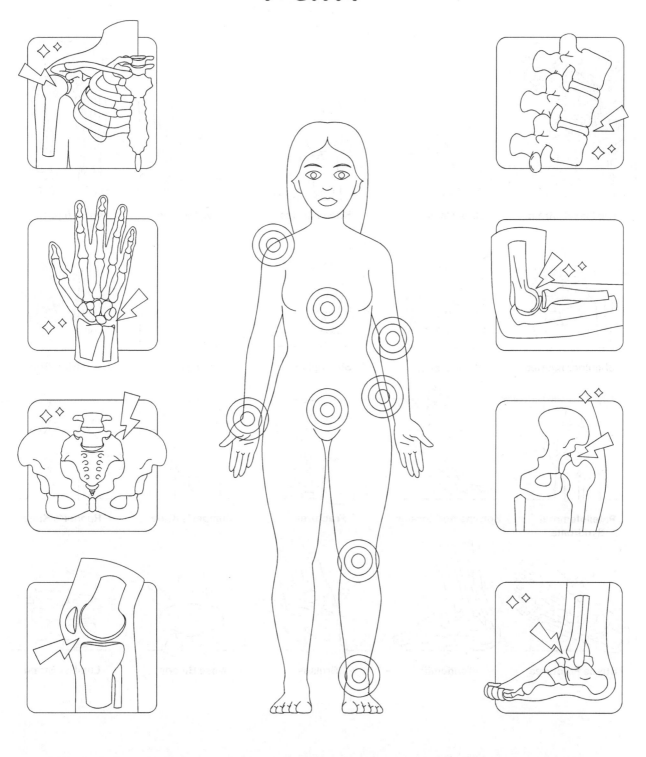

Sports Injuries

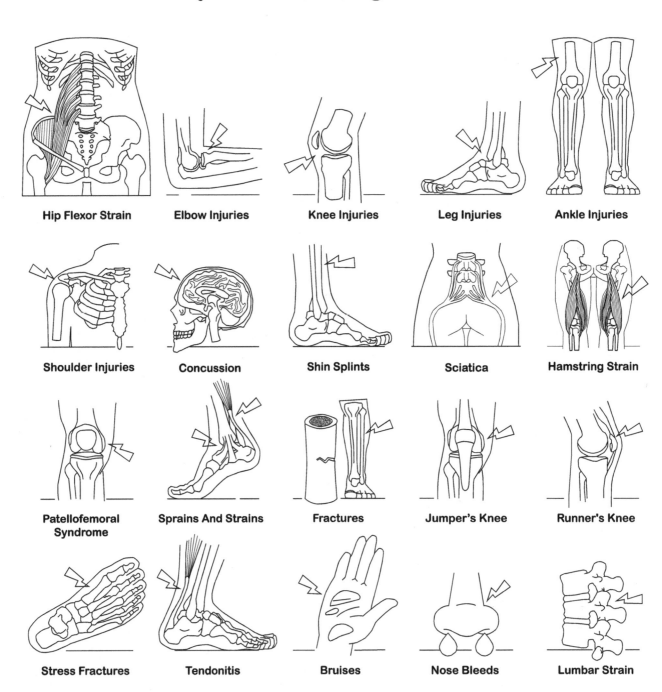

Hip Flexor Strain   Elbow Injuries   Knee Injuries   Leg Injuries   Ankle Injuries

Shoulder Injuries   Concussion   Shin Splints   Sciatica   Hamstring Strain

Patellofemoral Syndrome   Sprains And Strains   Fractures   Jumper's Knee   Runner's Knee

Stress Fractures   Tendonitis   Bruises   Nose Bleeds   Lumbar Strain

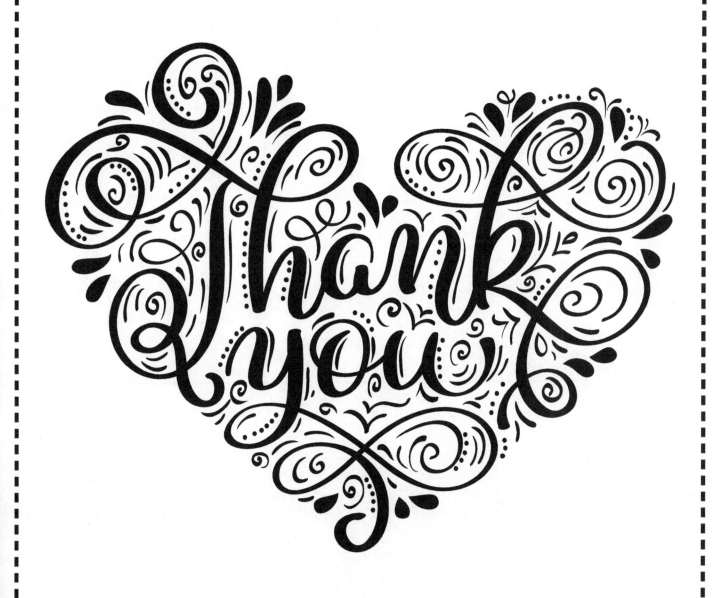

Made in United States
Troutdale, OR
11/16/2024

24887142R00053